POLICY AND PROCEDURAL GUIDELINES
FOR HYPERBARIC FACILITIES

OWEN J. O'NEILL, MD, MPH, FUHM
EDITOR

BEST PUBLISHING COMPANY

Copyright © 2017 Best Publishing Company

Printed and bound in the United States of America

ISBN: 978-1-947239-01-2
Library of Congress Catalog Number: 2017944120

Best Publishing Company
631 U.S. Highway 1, Suite 307
North Palm Beach, Florida 33408

TABLE OF CONTENTS

PATIENT CARE

HYPERBARIC CHAMBER

QUALITY IMPROVEMENT

APPENDICES

PREFACE

The field of hyperbaric medicine, along with hyperbaric centers throughout the United States and abroad, continues to grow. This growth has been exponential, touting an increase from 350 centers in 1993 to well over 2,500 programs today. With this progression exists a need to establish a resource guideline for developing complete and comprehensive policies and procedures for clinical hyperbaric units. Hyperbaric policy and procedures provide the guiding principles and foundation for safety, quality, transparency, and cost-effective hyperbaric medical and nursing practice. Every hyperbaric facility needs to follow its specific policies and procedures.

Policy and Procedural Guidelines for Hyperbaric Facilities provides needed resource and reference guidelines for new and established hyperbaric facilities. It will serve as a reference for the development of new hyperbaric policies as well as customize and enhance current policies and procedures already in place.

Policy and Procedural Guidelines for Hyperbaric Facilities addresses issues of safety and practice for both the multiplace and monoplace environments. It utilizes regulatory guidelines and standards of practice as its foundation. Topics covered in this work include, but are not limited to, governance, administration, emergency procedures, patient care, hyperbaric chamber maintenance, treatment protocols and quality improvement. The appendices include sample forms for both Class A multiplace and Class B monoplace chambers. They are intended to serve as templates for development of hyperbaric unit-specific forms. Also included are acronyms, references, and an index, all specific to hyperbaric medicine.

The guidelines provided in this document will benefit the diverse group of physicians, nurses, technicians, and allied health-care personnel in the hyperbaric field as they customize their unit-specific policies and procedures. The contributing authors are comprised of established experts in the field of undersea and hyperbaric medicine. They are a diverse group of physicians, nurses, and technologists who devoted an extensive amount of time and energy into producing this resource document of the highest quality. Specific acknowledgments can be found in a separate section of this book.

Owen J. O'Neill, MD, MPH, FUHM
Editor and Author

Laura Josefsen, RN, ACHRN
Contributing Author

LIST OF CONTRIBUTORS

Nick Bird, MD, MMM

Brock Chamberlain, CHT, DMT

Helen Gelly, MD, FUHM, FACCWS, UHM, ABPM

Bret Holliday, CHT

Laura Josefsen, RN, ACHRN, Contributing Author

Tracey Leigh LeGros, MD, PhD, FACEP, FAAEM, FUHM

Mitchell Mackey, EMT, CHT

Joann Marker, EMT, CHT

Heather Murphy-Lavoie, MD, FAAEM, FACEP, FUHM

Owen Joseph O'Neill, MD, MPH, FUHM, Contributing Author/Editor

Michael J. White, MD, MMM, UHM

W.T. Workman, MS, CAsP CHT-A, FASMA

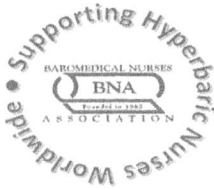

The Baromedical Nurses Association (established 1985) provides a forum for hyperbaric nursing that encompasses quality, safety, teamwork, mentoring, research, education, and nursing guidelines of standards of care for the patient receiving hyperbaric oxygen therapy.

The Baromedical Nurses Association endorses the *Policy and Procedural Guidelines for Hyperbaric Facilities* as guidelines to enable hyperbaric facilities to develop and/or expand their unit-specific policies.

GOVERNANCE

100 MISSION, VISION AND GOALS

The Hyperbaric Center

1.1 Mission

The mission is to provide an environment conducive to diagnosis and treatment with hyperbaric oxygen (HBO_2) therapy, as well as the education and support for patients, families and individuals responsible for the patient's care across all settings. Care is comprehensive, innovative, compassionate, cost-effective and shall focus on continuous improvement.

1.2 Vision

The vision of the Hyperbaric Center Program is to become the center of a network of community health-care resources for hyperbaric treatment according to Undersea and Hyperbaric Medical Society (UHMS) guidelines for approved indications.

1.3 Philosophy

The Hyperbaric Center Program provides care to patients, regardless of race, age, color, creed, sex, sexual orientation, national origin or handicap, providing individual inclusion criteria are met.

Patients and persons to the degree necessary or desirable by the patient (family members and/or those important to the patient) are significant members of the health-care team and have a right to participate in decision-making regarding their health-care regimen.

Quality health care will be delivered through open communication and collaboration with all members of the health-care team, regardless of discipline or setting.

1.4 Goals

The Hyperbaric Center Program, by way of a multidisciplinary approach to care and based on the holistic needs of the patient, is directed toward the following:

1.4.1 Achieving the highest quality care

1.4.2 Maintaining optimum levels of patient teaching/education

1.4.3 Utilizing state-of-the-art treatment that fosters and enhances quality of life

1.4.4 Obtaining optimal patient outcomes

101 CLINICAL STANDARDS

STANDARD I - Aspects of Care for Hyperbaric Treatments

Standards of Care

1.1 The patient shall have a competent, qualified, appropriately trained and credentialed hyperbaric physician, trained hyperbaric registered nurse and trained hyperbaric technologist responsible for planning, directing and providing his or her care.

    1.1.1 Training and credentialing should be appropriate for the type of chambers being used.

Standards of Practice

Practice standards will follow regulatory guidelines, evidence-practice research and current standard of practice for hyperbaric oxygen therapy.

1.2 Quality of Care

    1.2.1 Systematic evaluation of quality and efficacy of care

1.3 Performance Appraisal

    1.3.1 Conducted initially and annually

1.4 Clinical Staff Education

    1.4.1 Minimum requirement is a 40-hour approved introductory course in Undersea and Hyperbaric Medicine (UHM)

    1.4.2 Meets current mandatory and current industry-standard educational requirements

    1.4.3 Maintains current licensure and certification as appropriate

1.5 Collegiality

    1.5.1 Staff contributes to the professional development of peers, colleagues and others.

1.6 Collaboration

    1.6.1 Coordinates multidisciplinary aspects of care

1.7 Ethics

    1.7.1 Decisions are based on sound ethical practice.

1.8 Hyperbaric Research

    1.8.1 Staff participates in research activities as appropriate to the individual's

        1.8.1.1 Position

        1.8.1.2 Education

        1.8.1.3 Practice environment

STANDARD II - Environment

Standards of Care

2.1 The environment will be safe, clean, comfortable and therapeutic.

Standards of Practice

2.2 Equipment will be maintained per regulatory guidelines for both Class A multiplace and/or Class B monoplace chambers.

2.3 Infection control guidelines will follow established protocols for both Class A multiplace and/or Class B monoplace chambers.

2.4 Patient safety

    2.4.1 Safety guidelines meet or exceed industry standards.

STANDARD III - Assessment/Reassessment

Standards of Care

3.1 The patient shall be assessed for hyperbaric oxygen therapy by an appropriately trained and credentialed hyperbaric medicine physician and a trained hyperbaric nurse with experience commensurate for the types of chambers patients are being treated in.

Standards of Practice

3.2 The hyperbaric physician responsibility:

    3.2.1 Initial visit: timely and comprehensive patient consultation and assessment

    3.2.2 Patient reassessment on all subsequent hyperbaric treatments prior to entering and after exiting the chamber

STANDARD IV - Patient/Family and Caregiver Education

Standards of Care

4.1 The patient and/or person responsible for the patient's care shall be knowledgeable about the nature of the illness/wound, procedures and planned program directed toward health restoration and maintenance.

Standards of Practice

4.2 Education

    4.2.1 Education will be provided to patients and families.

    4.2.2. Ongoing education will be provided prior to every HBO_2 treatment and as the needs of the patient changes.

STANDARD V - Patient Rights

Standards of Care

5.1 The patient shall have a sense of acceptance as a person and of value as a human being and shall maintain a sense of personal identity.

Standards of Practice

5.2 Patient Care

    5.2.1 Patients will be approached and treated with respect.

    5.2.2 Open communication will be ongoing.

    5.2.3 Patients will be made aware of their rights.

102 HYPERBARIC SCOPE OF PRACTICE AND SERVICES

Purpose

1.1   To identify the scope of practice and services for the patient receiving hyperbaric oxygen therapy

1.2   The hyperbaric center staff qualifications and available equipment for providing hyperbaric oxygen therapy typically allow for the types of patients that are considered for treatment.

1.3   The hyperbaric center with qualified staff and available equipment may provide hyperbaric treatments for patients requiring:

    1.3.1   Ventilator support

    1.3.2   Continuous intravenous (IV) therapy

    1.3.3   Arterial lines

    1.3.4   Cardiac, hemodynamic or other invasive monitoring

1.4   Both Class A multiplace chambers and Class B monoplace chambers may provide these types of critical and urgent care needs with the appropriately trained physicians, nurses and technologists. All personnel who take part in these types of advanced treatment protocols must have appropriately documented training and experience.

Policy

2.1   Patients are treated using appropriate indications for hyperbaric oxygen therapy and within the scope of staff qualifications, available equipment and types of chambers (Class A or Class B).

    2.1.1   The hyperbaric physician will determine the patient qualification for hyperbaric treatment in accordance with the qualifications of the staff and availability of equipment.

2.2   Patients will receive hyperbaric oxygen therapy only when evaluated and ordered by a hyperbaric physician trained and credentialed in hyperbaric medicine with experience commensurate with the type of chambers being utilized (Class A or Class B).

2.3   The hyperbaric center shall not be a source of primary medical care.

Procedure

3.1   Patients will be evaluated by a physician trained and credentialed in hyperbaric oxygen therapy and a trained hyperbaric nurse prior to HBO_2 treatment and screened for appropriate diagnosis, relative and absolute contraindications to treatment, patient safety and the patients' underlying condition.

3.2   Patients and their HIPAA-compliant surrogates are encouraged to participate in the decision for HBO_2 therapy by receiving education regarding the risks and benefits and the expected outcomes of treatment and nontreatment of HBO_2 therapy. This should be delivered by the hyperbaric physician initially and reiterated by the hyperbaric team members as appropriate.

3.3   Physicians not trained and credentialed in HBO_2 therapy may request a referral or a consult to have a patient evaluated for HBO_2 therapy.

    3.3.1   The hyperbaric physician trained and credentialed in hyperbaric medicine

3.3.1.1 Will evaluate the patient

3.3.1.2 Determine the diagnosis and plan of care

3.3.1.3 Write the appropriate orders and oversee the hyperbaric oxygen treatments

3.4 A physician trained and credentialed in hyperbaric medicine will be immediately available during every hyperbaric patient treatment.

3.4.1 Physicians with Class B monoplace chambers should be readily available to handle hyperbaric emergencies and complications.

3.4.2 Physicians overseeing patients and team members working inside a Class A chamber should be present in the chamber room and immediately available to handle emergencies encountered with both patients and team members working inside the chamber.

3.4.3 Physicians working in Class A multiplace chamber settings should be cleared for exposure to extreme atmospheric environments and be able to enter the hyperbaric chamber to handle patient emergencies to the maximum depth of chamber capability.

3.5 A staff member trained in hyperbaric medicine, including completing at minimum, an approved 40-hour introductory course, will provide ongoing chamber-side monitoring during the patient HBO_2 treatment.

3.5.1 All staff members responsible for patient care and chamber operation should work toward becoming certified by the National Board of Diving and Hyperbaric Medical Technology (NBDHMT) and/or Baromedical Nurses Association Certification Board (BNACB).

3.5.2 All chamber operators of Class A multiplace chambers should be certified by the NBDHMT and/or BNACB and have appropriate training and experience.

3.5.3 All Class A multiplace chambers should have a minimum of one hyperbaric technologist certified by the NBDHMT and one hyperbaric nurse certified by BNACB on site during treatment hours and when chambers are compressed.

3.5.4 It is recommended that all hyperbaric facilities have one hyperbaric technologist and one hyperbaric nurse on site for daily treatments who are certified by the NBDHMT and/or BNACB.

3.6 The frequency and duration of HBO_2 treatments will depend upon the patient condition and treatment protocol per physician order.

3.7 Hyperbaric oxygen treatment schedules vary from center to center. Treatments are typically scheduled five days a week but may include a seven-days-a-week schedule including holidays. The patient's medical condition and diagnosis for requiring therapy guides the appropriate treatment schedule.

3.8 The hyperbaric unit normal hours of operation will be posted. After-hours' availability will also be stated on the voicemail message and will include contact information for emergent issues or general questions.

3.9 The hyperbaric physician will be in regular communication with the patient's primary care/referring physician.

3.10 Continuity of care is promoted through program integration across settings.

3.11 Emergent treatments will be at the discretion of the physician trained and credentialed in hyperbaric medicine and in accordance with staff qualifications, available equipment and types of chambers being utilized (Class A or Class B).

103 REGULATORY AGENCIES

Purpose

1.1 The hyperbaric center strives to meet or exceed the expectations of regulatory agencies (public and private) responsible for exercising authority or supervision.

Policy

2.1 The hyperbaric center staff will be aware of all regulatory agency guidelines for hyperbaric safety.

Procedure

3.1 The agencies overseeing various aspects of hyperbaric oxygen therapy include but are not limited to:

    3.1.1 ASME (American Society of Mechanical Engineers)

        3.1.1.1 Establishes the rules of safety for the design, fabrication and inspection of boilers and pressure vessels

        3.1.1.2 Consists of 11 sections

    3.1.2 PVHO-1 (Pressure Vessels for Human Occupancy)

        3.1.2.1 ASME Safety Standard

    3.1.3 ASTM (American Society for Testing and Materials)

        3.1.3.1 Provides testing for material safety in the hyperbaric environment

    3.1.4 CGA (Compressed Gas Association)

        3.1.4.1 Develops and promotes safety standards and safe practices in the industrial gas industry

    3.1.5 NFPA (National Fire Protection Association)

        3.1.5.1 Establishes criteria for levels of health care based on risk

    3.1.6 State and Local Authorities

104 STAFF TRAINING, EDUCATION AND COMPETENCIES

Purpose

1.1 Hyperbaric treatments require additional safety education and measures due to the altered environment of using 100% oxygen at increased atmospheric pressure.

1.2 The hyperbaric staff will receive mandatory training leading toward certification specific to hyperbaric medicine prior to working in the hyperbaric center.

1.3 The hyperbaric staff will receive appropriate and mandatory training commensurate with the types of chambers being utilized.

    1.3.1 Class B chamber staff will receive training commensurate with working with this type of equipment.

    1.3.2 Class A chamber staff will require appropriate training and experience commensurate with working inside extreme atmospheric pressure environments.

        1.3.2.1 Class A multiplace chambers are significantly more sophisticated and intricate in their operations. It is suggested that all hyperbaric physicians, nurses and technologists working in a Class A multiplace chamber environment meet the additional expected training and experience requirements.

Policy

2.1 The hyperbaric center will be staffed with adequate personnel whose qualifications are consistent with their job responsibilities and types of chambers utilized.

2.2 The validation of the hyperbaric staff education, training and competencies are the responsibility of the hyperbaric program director, hyperbaric medical director and the registered nurse manager.

Procedure

3.1 Initial competencies with documentation for all hyperbaric staff will be completed within 90 days of initial employment.

    3.1.1 Competencies will then be performed annually for all hyperbaric clinic staff.

    3.1.2 Current licensure and certification, including Basic Life Support, is to be maintained.

    3.1.3 All physicians and nurses should be advanced cardiac life support (ACLS) trained and certification maintained.

3.2 Staff Orientation and Education Requirements

    3.2.1 Physicians - All regular practitioners in the program who shall oversee the operation of the hyperbaric chamber shall have the following qualifications:

        3.2.1.1 Completion of a fellowship in UHM leading to board eligibility and/or board certification preferred.

        3.2.1.2 Physicians elected a Fellow in UHM are recognized as national and international leaders in the field of UHM.

3.2.1.3 Completion of a formal UHM-approved 40-hour hyperbaric introductory course with 40 hours exclusively devoted to hyperbaric medicine theory and practice and successful completion of the course examination is acceptable.

3.2.1.4 Board certification or board eligible in the physician's primary specialty if other than hyperbaric medicine in addition to the 40-hour course requirement.

3.2.1.5 Board certification in UHM is strongly encouraged.

3.2.1.6 Ongoing education in hyperbaric medicine practice is strongly encouraged.

3.2.1.7 Experience must be commensurate with the type of hyperbaric chambers being utilized. Physicians working in Class A chambers for the first time must be mentored by a hyperbaric physician whose Class A chamber experience is not less than two years or who has successfully completed an accredited UHM fellowship training program. Mentorship should be for a period of not less than six months and may be extended by the mentor if more training time is considered necessary, especially pertaining to understanding dive tables, repetitive dive tables, mixed gas tables and the mitigation of decompression sickness of the inside observers. Physicians are expected to enter the hyperbaric chamber to handle emergencies and assist with chamber operations if and when necessary.

3.2.2 Registered Nurse and Technician Requirements

3.2.2.1 Complete a formal UHM-approved 40-hour hyperbaric introductory course.

3.2.2.2 The safety director will additionally complete a safety director course approved by the NBDHMT and have the experience commensurate with the types of chambers being utilized by the center (Class A and/or Class B).

3.2.2.3 Hyperbaric clinical personnel (nurses and technicians) are to achieve hyperbaric certification when eligible and preferably within two years of being employed.

3.2.2.4 Ongoing education in hyperbaric medicine practice is strongly encouraged and necessary for maintenance of certification by certain boards and societies.

3.2.3 New personnel, full time, part time, and per diem, will receive orientation of sufficient duration and content to prepare them for their specific duties and responsibilities.

3.2.4 It is preferred that hyperbaric staff not certified by the NBDHMT and/or BNACB should be overseen by certified staff.

3.2.5 The Hyperbaric Center Program shall cooperate with the hospital facility education department in providing an initial hospital orientation program for all personnel and in the provision of ongoing in-service or continuing education programs. These programs are designed to augment the staff and community of pertinent new developments in hyperbaric patient care and to maintain current competence.

3.3 The hyperbaric facility staff are encouraged to participate in seminars, workshops and other educational activities related to the practice of hyperbaric medicine and facility safety.

3.3.1 The hyperbaric facility staff may submit requests to attend and participate in seminars, workshops and other educational activities related to the practice of hyperbaric medicine and facility safety.

3.3.2 Approval will be dependent upon available education funding, facility staffing and procedure related to these activities.

3.4 A hyperbaric reference library will be accessible to all hyperbaric facility staff.

105 HYPERBARIC TEACHING AND PUBLISHING

Purpose

1.1 To ensure that publications and marketing materials meet the standards and clinical, information, regulatory, and security guidelines of the hospital facility and the UHMS

1.2 To determine the information presented accurately reflects scope of service

Policy

2.1 The hyperbaric facility and appropriate hyperbaric administration will approve all publications, including but not limited to policies, marketing, educational presentations, brochures, articles, pamphlets, and scientific publications attributed to the hyperbaric center.

Procedure

3.1 All publications will be presented to the appropriate hyperbaric administration for approval prior to publication or presentation.

3.2 Policies, procedures, courses, copies of abstracts, articles, scientific papers, etc., published or presented by staff members will be available in the department for a minimum of three years prior to an accreditation survey and for review by interested parties, either written and/or electronic.

3.3 Copies of all course control documents (plan of instructions, etc.) for courses taught by the staff of the hyperbaric facility will be available for a minimum of three years prior to an accreditation survey.

3.4 Copies of all documents submitted to the UHMS or to the NBDHMT for course review and approval will be available for a minimum of three years prior to an accreditation survey for review by the accreditation team, if requested.

3.5 All marketing materials will be limited to reflect the scope of practice of the wound care and hyperbaric unit.

3.6 The staff of the wound care and hyperbaric facility are encouraged to be actively involved in the medical and lay community educational activities related to research and to the practice of wound care and hyperbaric medicine through educational presentations and marketing.

   3.6.1 Whenever possible, staff will be relieved from direct patient care and administrative activities to enable participation in research, medical and lay community education and marketing.

106 CLINICAL RESEARCH

Purpose

1.1 Clinical research at the HBO_2 facility will be performed per regulatory Institutional Review Board (IRB) guidelines.

Policy

2.1 Clinical research will be conducted only upon approval of an IRB.

2.2 Clinical research conducted in the hyperbaric facility will be appropriate to the expertise and qualifications of the staff and resources of the facility.

Procedure

3.1 All clinical research will be in accordance with IRB research protocols.

3.2 Clinical research will be performed in accordance with ethical and professional practice and legal requirements.

3.3 Clinical research will be periodically monitored.

3.4 Personnel involved in clinical research will have adequate facilities to do the research.

3.5 Provisions are made to ensure the rights and welfare of all research subjects are adequately protected.

3.6 The informed consent for the clinical research will be in English, as well as in the language spoken by the subject.

3.7 The informed consent is obtained by adequate and appropriate methods.

3.8 Patients receiving hyperbaric treatments involved in research are informed of:

    3.8.1 The research project having IRB approval

    3.8.2 Description of the benefits, risks and procedures

    3.8.3 Refusal to participate will not compromise their access to hyperbaric treatments.

ADMINISTRATION

200 ADMINISTRATION PROGRAM

Purpose

1.1 To ensure the Hyperbaric Center Program runs smoothly and professionally within the appropriate hospital setting

Policy

2.1 The hyperbaric center shall support the mission, philosophy, goals and objectives of the hospital facility, as well as meeting or exceeding the criteria for hyperbaric treatment as established by regulatory, accreditation and supervising agencies both public and private.

2.2 The department director prepares a capital equipment budget annually and according to directives provided by the hospital administration.

Procedure

3.1 Provide for safety in a specialized environment.

3.2 Provide comprehensive, integrated services.

3.3 Provide an educational framework for patients and staff.

3.4 Promote the involvement of patient and family members in the decisions regarding health care and health-care alternatives.

3.5 Provide a systematic and ongoing performance improvement program.

3.6 Maintain qualified and competent staff through provision of education, training and competency verification on a regular basis.

3.7 Provide a program of community awareness regarding the scope of the program's services for both the internal and external communities.

3.8 Hyperbaric Center Meetings

    3.8.1 Physician Staff Meeting (quarterly)

    3.8.2 Peer Review Team Conference (monthly and as indicated)

    3.8.3 Department Staff Meeting (monthly)

    3.8.4 Staff Performance Improvement Committee (monthly)

    3.8.5 Policy and Procedure Committee (annually)

3.9 Recommended Hyperbaric Staff Involvement in Hospital Facility Meetings

    3.9.1 Hospital Safety Committee

    3.9.2 Quality Improvement Committee

3.10 Minutes are recorded for all committee and staff meetings and are circulated and/or reviewed with staff.

POLICY AND PROCEDURAL GUIDELINES FOR HYPERBARIC FACILITIES
Copyright © 2017 Best Publishing Company

201 POLICY AND PROCEDURE GUIDELINES

Purpose

1.1 *Policy and Procedural Guidelines for Hyperbaric Facilities* will be used to supplement the hospital facility policies and procedures for clinical practice in the hyperbaric center to meet safety and regulatory guidelines.

Policy

2.1 The hyperbaric center will practice per policies and procedures as set forth by the hospital facility and additionally by *Policy and Procedural Guidelines for Hyperbaric Facilities.*

2.2 *Policy and Procedural Guidelines for Hyperbaric Facilities* is intended to provide a basis for developing unit-specific hyperbaric policies and procedures that are to be used as a supplement to the hospital facility policy and procedure manual.

2.2.1 The hospital facility will review and agree with the unit-specific policies and procedures.

2.3 A hard copy of the hyperbaric specific policies and procedures will be located in the hyperbaric center.

2.4 Hyperbaric-specific policies and procedures are revised/reviewed annually.

Procedure

3.1 Hyperbaric staff will be familiar with the hyperbaric-specific policies.

3.2 Hyperbaric staff will be notified of new or revised policies.

3.3 Hyperbaric staff will be notified when they are not compliant with hyperbaric policy and procedures and be given a specified time to rectify the noncompliance.

202 MEDICAL RECORD RETENTION

Purpose

1.1 Medical records furnish documentary evidence of the course of care given to patients.

1.2 It is the intent of the hyperbaric center to safeguard the record and the confidentiality of its contents at all times.

Policy

2.1 The hyperbaric center will adhere to all federal, state, and local laws concerning medical record retention and confidentiality.

2.2 The hyperbaric center will follow the hospital guidelines for retention and storage of records.

2.3 The minimum retention period for the medical record chart is governed by the site hospital facility state statute.

Procedure

3.1 Medical records should be stored in compliance with state and federal regulations and be locked in a secure area when the unit is closed.

3.2 Electronic medical records are password protected.

3.3 Medical records are to be kept confidential and where patients may not view the information for any other patient.

3.4 Only appropriate health-care personnel are allowed to document in the patient record.

203 BILLING DOCUMENTATION

Purpose

1.1 To ensure continuity of care and complete documentation

1.2 To meet compliance with hospital, state, federal, UHMS, The Joint Commission (TJC), Centers for Medicare and Medicaid Services (CMS) and regulatory guidelines

Policy

2.1 Documentation for hyperbaric medicine is to meet or exceed hospital, state, CMS, private industry and TJC requirements.

Procedure

3.1 Documentation is the tool used to validate medical and nursing practice.

3.2 The following are to be considered when reviewing documentation:

   3.2.1 State regulations

   3.2.2 Federal regulations

   3.2.3 Accreditation agencies

   3.2.4 Hospital policies

   3.2.5 Corporate policies

   3.2.6 Professional organizations

   3.2.7 Reimbursement (Approved conditions must be determined to meet medical necessity.)

   3.2.8 Approved diagnosis and procedure codes

   3.2.9 Documentation in place to support diagnosis

   3.2.10 Supporting documentation for any billed service

   3.2.11 Documented physician order in place for any service

   3.2.12 Informed consent in place for procedures and hyperbaric oxygen treatments

3.3 Medical records should include:

   3.3.1 Changes in patient condition, treatment, medication and wound

   3.3.2 Daily complete detailed HBO_2 treatment

   3.3.3 Physician progress notes

   3.3.4 Comprehensive patient assessment

   3.3.5 Patient-specific plan of care - medical and nursing

3.3.6 Procedures, ancillary equipment, dates and times

3.3.7 Medication list and reconciliation report, initial and ongoing

3.3.8 Patient-specific initial and ongoing outcomes and goals

3.3.9 Education plans and evidence of teaching

3.3.10 Signed physician orders - dated and timed

3.3.11 Coordination of services

3.3.12 Discharge planning

204 PATIENT ACCEPTANCE FOR HYPERBARIC OXYGEN TREATMENT

Purpose

1.1 Due to the safety issues involved with hyperbaric oxygen therapy, the patients receiving hyperbaric oxygen therapy must be evaluated by a physician trained and credentialed in hyperbaric medicine to decrease the potential for adverse events while receiving hyperbaric oxygen treatment.

Policy

2.1 Patients will receive hyperbaric oxygen therapy upon evaluation by a trained and credentialed hyperbaric physician with the appropriate and documented experience commensurate with the types of chambers utilized by the facility (Class A or Class B).

Procedure

3.1 Patients will be accepted for hyperbaric oxygen therapy following:

   3.1.1 Acceptance of a patient from a referring physician or facility, or self-referred, after direct communication with and acceptance by the hyperbaric physician of record.

   3.1.2 Medical information will be requested from physicians who have participated in the patient's care following a medical release form signed by the patient. The administrative assistant or staff nurse will request the medical information upon request of the hyperbaric physician.

   3.1.3 Timely pretreatment evaluation of any patient for HBO_2 therapy after notification of a consult request has been received by the center.

   3.1.4 The trained and credentialed hyperbaric physician performing the consult shall order HBO_2 therapy and any other services appropriate to the patient's disease and or condition, if the patient is qualified.

   3.1.5 The hyperbaric center physician shall communicate with the patient's referring and/or primary physician with regard to acceptance of the patient to include progress of the therapy in a timely fashion.

   3.1.6 Hyperbaric oxygen therapy shall be available to accepted patients as deemed necessary by the hyperbaric trained and credentialed physician of record and/or the center's hyperbaric-trained and credentialed medical director.

   3.1.7 Hyperbaric oxygen therapy shall be performed only after the hyperbaric physician consult and an appropriate informed consent form for treatment has been signed and dated by the physician, patient, or patient's representative. The consult should be documented and made available to the hyperbaric center with the appropriate hyperbaric and supporting documentation.

   3.1.8 The hyperbaric physician shall provide the written orders for the hyperbaric treatments.

   3.1.9 During the course of therapy at the hyperbaric center, any monitoring or medication deemed necessary shall be prescribed to the patients provided by qualified personnel in accordance accepted medical practice.

3.1.10 During the course of therapy, patients may be referred to other hospital-based services, including but not limited to:

3.1.10.1 Diabetes education

3.1.10.2 Home health agency

3.1.10.3 Imaging

3.1.10.4 Laboratory

3.1.10.5 Nutritional counseling

3.1.10.6 Occupational/rehabilitative medicine

3.1.10.7 Surgical services

3.1.11 Physician attendance will be in place during hyperbaric treatments, minimally per UHMS and CMS guidelines and those specific for each center depending on the types of chambers utilized (Class A or Class B or both).

3.1.11.1 Minimal standard for physician attendance during treatment in Class B chambers is during compression and decompression phases.

3.1.11.2 Class A chamber physician attendance should be continual for the entire treatment.

3.1.12 Patient shall be discharged by written order from the hyperbaric physician of record in a time frame determined by and acceptable to the hyperbaric center.

205 MISSED APPOINTMENTS

Purpose

1.1 To establish guidelines for the management of patients who have missed one or more appointments with the center

Policy

2.1 Management of patients who miss one or more appointments shall be handled by designated personnel according to the following procedures.

Procedure

3.1 When a patient misses several regular appointments or a final discharge appointment and does not call the center to reschedule, the nursing case manager shall:

   3.1.1 Notify the hyperbaric physician of record.

   3.1.2 Call the patient the same day as the scheduled appointment, determine reason the patient missed the appointment, and reschedule the appointment as appropriate.

   3.1.3 Document the communication with the patient (telephone call) in the patient's chart.

   3.1.4 If unable to reach the patient by telephone (calls attempted by hyperbaric physician of record, office assistant and the case manager) a Missed Appointment Letter shall be mailed to the patient by certified mail/receipt requested, copied to the hyperbaric physician of record and the primary/referring physician.

   3.1.5 Documentation in the patient medical record will show the letter was sent, a copy placed in the chart, and shall include the certified mail/receipt confirmation number.

3.2 When a patient does not respond to the Missed Appointment Letter, the case manager shall:

   3.2.1 Have the hyperbaric physician of record mail a Self-Discharge Against Medical Advice Letter to the patient within two weeks from the mailing date of the case manager letter (certified mail/receipt requested), copied to the primary/referring physician.

   3.2.2 Place a copy of the Self-Discharge Against Medical Advice Letter in the patient's chart.

3.3 When a patient does not respond to the Self-Discharge Against Medical Advice Letter within two weeks from the mailing date, the case manager shall:

   3.3.1 Have the center physician write and sign the Self-Discharge Against Medical Advice in the patient's chart.

   3.3.2 Discharge the patient from the center after the Self-Discharge Against Medical Advice order has been written in the patient's chart and confirmed by the nurse case manager - notify patient's primary/referring physician.

   3.3.3 The case manager shall be responsible for:

      3.3.3.1 Reviewing the patient compliance list on a weekly basis.

3.3.3.2 Discuss noncompliance with the hyperbaric physician of record and the department medical director to determine appropriate action.

3.3.3.3 Document actions taken for missed appointments. The department director along with the case manager shall review this process on a quarterly basis and document the status.

3.4 When a patient calls and reschedules an appointment three or more times, the department director shall:

3.4.1 Evaluate the patient's compliance.

3.4.2 Refer the patient's status to the hyperbaric physician of record and/or the medical director. The hyperbaric physician of record or medical director shall speak with the patient directly or send a letter to the patient if necessary and communicate the results to the hyperbaric director or manager.

206 INCIDENT REPORTS

Purpose

1.1 An incident is defined as any unplanned event that may lead to potential harm to patients, staff or visitors.

Policy

2.1 Employees are to report any incident no matter how seemingly trivial that affects or may have affected the safety of an employee, patient, or visitor.

Procedure

3.1 Incident report forms shall be located in a designated location in a binder labeled "Incident Reports" if not available electronically.

3.2 The incident report form may be obtained from the hospital facility, or if not available from there, it will be in the hyperbaric center.

3.3 The employee MUST report any incident immediately to the hospital director of human resources, hyperbaric program director, safety director, physician and nurse manager.

3.4 Document the information immediately. Keep in mind that memory for detail fades quickly, and the most accurate information is documented immediately.

3.5 All areas of the incident report form MUST be completed. If the area does not relate to your incident, "N/A" may be used to ensure the area was addressed and is not filled in at a later date.

3.6 Careful attention should be paid to time, place, witnesses and details of the incident.

3.7 Handwriting MUST be legible.

   3.7.1 In your own words, describe what happened.

   3.7.2 Include in your report incident, complications, if any, equipment involved, when, where, who, and witnesses while avoiding hearsay.

3.8 The employee will be instructed by the hyperbaric program director where to report for evaluation of injury.

3.9 The employee must report for evaluation any injury or incident when instructed.

3.10 Depending on the incident and the circumstances surrounding it, the employee may be subject to drug testing when deemed necessary.

3.11 For the employee adverse event, this reporting is necessary even if no loss of work is anticipated.

3.12 For patient or visitor adverse event, evaluate whether the patient or visitor needs to be transferred to the emergency department.

   3.12.1 Document evaluation, treatment, follow-up treatment, and, as appropriate, notify health-care personnel, i.e., primary/referring physician, patient's family, etc. per hospital policy.

207 VISITORS IN THE HYPERBARIC CENTER

Purpose

1.1 The unique environment of the hyperbaric facility results in specific limitations for visitors to ensure patient, staff, and visitor safety, to decrease the potential for breach of patient information, and to safeguard patient privacy.

Policy

2.1 The hyperbaric center will follow the hospital facility visitor policy. This policy is to supplement the hospital facility policy for the specific issues of the hyperbaric center.

2.2 Visitation will be allowed at the discretion of the hyperbaric unit clinical staff.

    2.2.1 Specific permission will be required by the hyperbaric staff and the patient.

    2.2.2 Patient privacy will be respected.

2.3 Infection control standards will be maintained.

2.4 Children under the age of 12 are not allowed in the hyperbaric treatment area during patient care or treatment.

2.5 Photographs taken by visitors will be allowed only with the written prior authorization stating approval.

Procedure

Visitors are encouraged to visit the hyperbaric room under the following guidelines:

3.1 Specific permission by the hyperbaric staff and patient will be obtained for visitors coming into the hyperbaric treatment room.

3.2 Privacy of patient care will be respected.

3.3 Photographs taken by visitors/family members will only be allowed with prior written authorization stating approval by the hyperbaric staff and the patient.

3.4 HIPAA compliance will be followed.

3.5 At the patient request, a family member may accompany the patient to a patient care area as long as privacy of other patients is respected.

3.6 Visitors with illnesses (including respiratory infections) or draining infected wounds are not allowed in patient care areas.

3.7 Children under the age of 12 are not allowed in the hyperbaric treatment area during patient care or treatment.

3.8 Infection control standards will be maintained for visitors as well as clinical staff.

208 HYPERBARIC INDICATIONS

Purpose

1.1 The Hyperbaric Oxygen Therapy Committee of the UHMS reviews research, clinical data, and evidence that is regularly updated and published in the *UHMS Hyperbaric Oxygen Therapy Indications* manual.

1.2 The Hyperbaric Oxygen Therapy Committee of the UHMS reviews research, clinical data and evidence, which includes the following: sound physiologic rationale; in vivo or in vitro studies to demonstrate effectiveness; controlled animal studies; prospective controlled clinical studies; and extensive clinical experience from multiple, recognized hyperbaric medicine centers. This information is updated regularly and published in *UHMS Hyperbaric Oxygen Therapy Indications* manual.

1.3 Many of the following indications have an emergent as well as a non-emergent component.

Policy

Routine hyperbaric oxygen treatments will generally follow the accepted indications of the UHMS guidelines. Treatments may be considered elective, urgent, or emergent. Thus, the appropriate training and experience should be commensurate with the type of treatments being performed and the types of chambers being utilized (Class A or Class B chambers).

2.1 Indications for Hyperbaric Oxygen Treatments [1-14]

Hyperbaric oxygen therapy indications and treatment protocols are described in detail in the *UHMS Hyperbaric Oxygen Therapy Indications* manual. Please refer to the manual for full details and treatment recommendations.

2.1.1 Air or Gas Embolism

2.1.2 Arterial Insufficiencies

    2.1.2.1 Central Retinal Artery Occlusion

    2.1.2.2 Enhancement of Healing in Selected Problem

2.1.3 Carbon Monoxide Poisoning

2.1.4 Clostridial Myonecrosis (Gas Gangrene)

2.1.5 Compromised Grafts and Flaps

2.1.6 Crush Injuries and Skeletal Muscle-Compartment Syndromes

2.1.7 Decompression Sickness

2.1.8 Delayed Radiation Injuries (Soft Tissue and Bony Necrosis)

2.1.9 Idiopathic Sudden Sensorineural Hearing Loss

2.1.10 Intracranial Abscess

2.1.11 Necrotizing Soft Tissue Infections

2.1.12 Refractory Osteomyelitis

2.1.13 Severe Anemia

2.1.14 Thermal Burns

Procedure

The hyperbaric physician prescribes hyperbaric oxygen treatments and dosing, typically from 2.0-3.0 ATA (atmosphere absolute). Typical oxygen dosing is 90 minutes, divided into 30-minute oxygen breathing periods separated by 5-minute air breaks. Oxygen dosing and air breaks may vary at the discretion of the hyperbaric physician, depending on the type and availability of equipment, the patient's overall clinical condition and diagnosis. The following are guidelines for physicians to consider for hyperbaric treatment. (For full details and treatment options, please refer to *UHMS Hyperbaric Oxygen Therapy Indications* manual.)

3.1 Air or Gas Embolism[1]

    3.1.1 Recommended treatment protocols vary depending on physician expertise and available resources.

    3.1.2 USN Treatment Table 6 or equivalent

    3.1.3 Deeper tables or extending the number of oxygen breathing periods may be considered, depending on the physician's expertise and available resources, including number of employees and types of equipment.

    3.1.4 Utilization review is recommended following 10 treatments.

3.2 Carbon Monoxide Poisoning (CO)[3]

While some hyperbaric centers treat with a single HBO_2 session at the discretion of the medical director, treating physician or specific center policy, the best evidence for reduced cognitive sequelae after CO poisoning is to use 3 HBO_2 treatments within 24 hours. Recommend HBO_2 treatments 3 times within 24 hours. Class A and B chambers may initially compress to 3 ATA, then 2 ATA for 140 minutes, followed by 2 HBO_2 sessions at 2 ATA for 90 minutes (5-minute air breathing periods were used periodically to reduce oxygen toxicity) in 6- to 12-hour intervals. Initial compression to 2.8 ATA, then 2 ATA for 120 minutes, without further HBO_2.

    3.2.1 CO poisoning complicated by cyanide poisoning

    3.2.2 HBO_2 is recommended as an adjunct to the treatment of combined CO poisoning complicated by cyanide poisoning.

        3.2.2.1 Utilization review has not been well delineated.

3.3 Clostridial Myositis and Myonecrosis (Gas Gangrene)[4]

    3.3.1 HBO_2 is used in combination with surgery and antibiotic therapy.

        3.3.1.1. Coordinate with surgeon and surgery schedule.

3.3.1.2 Recommend 3 treatments within the first 24 hours. Provide at least a two-hour surface interval, preferably four hours between treatments to decrease risk of pulmonary oxygen toxicity. Treatment 1 should be at 3.0 ATA followed by standard wound healing treatments at 2-2.4 ATA.

3.3.1.3 Administer twice-a-day treatments for the next 2-5 days at 2-2.4 ATA.

3.3.2 Utilization review is indicated after 10 treatments.

3.4 Crush Injury, Compartment Syndrome and other Acute Traumatic Ischemias[6]

3.4.1 Treatment may vary from 2.0-2.4 ATA. Treatment duration will be 90-120 minutes, depending on treatment depth chosen and extent of injury. Treatments should be initiated twice daily on Day 1 and continue twice daily for up to 10 days depending on the severity of the ischemia, need for fasciotomy, extent of fasciotomy, clinical response and stabilization of the ischemia by clinical examination, testing and physician collaboration.

3.4.2 Utilization review: Crush injury and compartment syndrome initiated by hyperbaric physician through collaboration with the trauma/orthopedic surgeon, plastic/reconstructive surgeon and/or primary care physician.

3.4.2.1 Recommended after three treatments for impending stage of compartment syndrome

3.4.2.2 Recommended after 7 days or 14 HBO_2 treatments for managing post-fasciotomy site where the grafts or flaps are threatened

3.4.2.3 HBO_2 should be instituted if subsequent skin grafting or delayed closure is done for the fasciotomy site, and the graft or flaps are threatened.

3.5 Decompression Sickness[7]

3.5.1 Hyperbaric protocols for treating decompression sickness can vary significantly, and treatments are dictated per usual protocols, physician experience and patient response. Hyperbaric physicians should have broad knowledge of decompression schedules and be significantly experienced with their use. Decompression schedules should be on hand and easily accessible for reference. Typical recommendations are as follows:

3.5.1.1 Use USN Treatment Table 5 for Type I DCS at the discretion of the treating physician.

3.5.1.2 Use USN Treatment Table 6 for Type I or Type II DCS at the discretion of the treating physician.

3.5.1.3 Oxygen extension periods may be considered at the discretion of the hyperbaric physician.

3.5.1.4 USNTT 6A may be considered for extreme circumstances utilizing a Class A chamber. The hyperbaric physician and staff should be properly trained and experienced with the appropriate dive decompression schedules and mixed gas knowledge if and when mixed gases are utilized for decompression of patients and inside observers.

3.5.1.5 Utilization review is recommended after 10 treatments.

NOTE: Treatments performed subsequent to the initial TT6 or equivalent may include a repeat of TT6, TT5 or standard wound care treatments. The choice of treatment table used as well as the frequency of treatment will depend on the patient's condition and operational capacity of the department. If symptoms are not completely resolved but remain stable following repetitive USN TT5 or TT6, significant consideration must be given to alternative (differential) diagnoses that produce symptoms similar to decompression sickness. Once all differential diagnoses have been considered, repetitive or tailing treatments may be considered once or twice a day until symptoms are resolved or until no further improvement occurs. Tailing treatments are considered controversial despite a tendency to demonstrate improvement in certain cases. Treatments are performed at variable depths and times and are at the discretion of the hyperbaric physician properly trained and experienced in diving medicine. Treatments may be discontinued at the hyperbaric physician's determination when the tailing treatments have not resulted in patient improvement and the patient's symptoms have plateaued.

3.5.2 Altitude Decompression Sickness

3.5.2.1 Symptoms that clear on descent to ground level with normal neurological exam: 100% oxygen by tightly fitted mask for 2 hours minimum; aggressive oral hydration; observe 24 hours.

3.5.2.2 Symptoms that persist after return to ground level or occur at ground level: 100% oxygen; aggressive hydration; hyperbaric treatment using U.S. Navy Treatment Tables 5 or 6 as appropriate.

3.5.2.3 For individuals with symptoms consisting only of limb pain that resolves during oxygen breathing while preparing for hyperbaric treatment, a 24-hour period of observation should be initiated; hyperbaric therapy may not be required.

3.5.2.4 For severe symptoms of DCS including neurological symptoms, "chokes," hypotension or symptoms that progress in intensity despite oxygen therapy: continue 100% oxygen; administer intravenous hydration; and initiate immediate hyperbaric therapy using U.S. Navy Treatment Table 6.

3.5.2.5 Utilization review should occur after 10 treatments.

3.6 Arterial Insufficiencies[2a-2b]

3.6.1 Central Retinal Artery Occlusion - suggested HBO_2 treatment guidelines:

3.6.1.1 Deliver oxygen immediately at 1 ATA at the highest possible fraction of inspired oxygen (FiO_2).

3.6.1.2 If vision improves significantly with normobaric oxygen within 15 minutes, the patient should be admitted to the hospital and given intermittent normobaric oxygen for 15 minutes every hour, alternating with 45 minutes of breathing room air. Visual acuity should be checked at the end of each air-breathing period. This regimen should be continued until a fluorescein angiogram shows patency, the patient's vision remains stable on room air for 2 hours or a maximum time of 96 hours on intermittent supplemental oxygen therapy has been reached.

3.6.1.3 Refer for emergent hyperbaric oxygen therapy if no response within the first 15 minutes.

3.6.1.4 Compress to 2 ATA on 100% oxygen. Other adjunctive therapies to lower intraocular pressure and/or cause retinal vasodilatation may be performed as well but should not delay compression. If vision improves significantly at 2 ATA, remain at this depth for 90 minutes (air-breathing periods at this depth may not be necessary since the incidence of oxygen toxicity seizures is 4 times lower at 2 ATA than at 2.4 ATA.) Then proceed as outlined in section 3.6.1.7.

3.6.1.5 If vision fails to improve significantly at 2 ATA by the first air-breathing period (or 30 minutes), compress to 2.4 ATA. If vision improves significantly at this depth, conduct a U.S. Navy Treatment Table 9 and then proceed as outlined in 3.6.1.7 below.

3.6.1.6 If vision does not improve significantly at 2.4 ATA, compress to 2.8 ATA. If no improvement occurs after the first 20-minute breathing period, consider conducting a U.S. Navy Treatment Table 6. If vision improves significantly, proceed as outlined in 3.6.1.7 below. If there is no response to the initial Table 6 treatment, options are to discontinue treatment, continue with normobaric oxygen as in 3.6.1.2 or give 2 additional treatments for 90 minutes at 2.8 ATA with air-breathing periods on a twice-daily schedule.

3.6.1.7 If the patient has return of vision during hyperbaric treatment, inpatient monitoring and intermittent supplemental oxygen should be considered. Monitoring by a retina specialist should continue. Recovery of vision during the initial treatment of CRAO with HBO_2 indicates retinal viability and the potential for return of vision despite the ischemic period suffered prior to treatment. Patients with such a recovery should have their visual status monitored frequently after completion of HBO_2.

3.6.1.8 The majority of patients will stabilize within one week of symptom onset.

3.6.1.9 Utilization review recommended for patients treated for more than three days after clinical plateau and no further improvement.

3.6.2 Enhancement of Healing in Selected Problem Wounds

3.6.2.1 Diabetic lower extremity wounds

3.6.2.1.1 Patient has controlled Type 1 or 2 diabetes, nonreconstructible vascular disease and a lower extremity wound.

3.6.2.1.2 Wound is classified as a Wagner Grade 3 or higher.

3.6.2.1.3 Patient has failed an adequate course of standard wound therapy for 30 days and documented nonreconstructible vascular disease by a qualified vascular surgeon.

3.6.2.2 Utilization review required after the initial 30 days of treatment and at least that frequently thereafter.

3.7 Acute Traumatic Peripheral Ischemias (ATPI)[2a-2b]

3.7.1 Treatment with hyperbaric oxygen is similar to treatment protocol for ATPI.

3.7.2 HBO_2 treatments are delivered at 2–2.5 ATA for 90 to 120 minutes of oxygen breathing once or twice daily.

3.7.3 Utilization review is also similar to ATPI. Utilization review should be performed after the initial 30 days of treatment and at least that frequently thereafter.

3.8 Severe and Refractory Anemia[13]

This is the inability of certain patients to accept blood transfusions for any reason, the most common based on religious beliefs. Untoward inflammatory and immunomodulatory effects of large red blood cell (RBC) transfusions may also be a reason to seek alternatives to transfusion.

3.8.1 Pulsed HBO_2 may be effective in reducing oxygen debt in severe anemia.

3.8.2 Treatments can be delivered at 2.0-3.0 ATA for 3- to 4-hour treatment times, 3 to 4 times per day with appropriate air breaks to decrease risk of oxygen toxicity.

3.8.3 Treatment may be continued until the RBC have been replaced adequately by patient regeneration or eventual acceptance of transfusion.

3.9 Intracranial Abscess[10]

3.9.1 HBO_2 is considered when there are multiple abscesses in a deep or dominant location, compromised hosts, fungal abscesses, or where surgery is contraindicated and there is minimal response to usual measures.

3.9.2 Treatment is initiated at pressures from 2.0-2.5 ATA, 100% oxygen for 60-90 minutes daily.

3.9.3 Twice-daily treatments may be considered appropriate pending the patient's overall condition and treatment tolerance.

3.9.4 Utilization review is suggested after 20 treatments.

3.10 Necrotizing Soft Tissue Infections[11]

3.10.1 HBO_2 is an adjunct treatment to surgical debridement, antibiotic therapy.

3.10.2 Treatments are initiated at 2.0-2.4 ATA for 90 minutes twice daily for infections other than clostridial necrosis.

3.10.3 Clostridial necrosis and myonecrosis should be treated at increased pressures 2.8-3.0 ATA with gas gangrene protocol in the first 24 hours, then twice daily until patient is stable as evidenced by nonprogression of necrosis.

3.10.4 Utilization review should be requested after 30 treatments.

3.11 Osteomyelitis (Refractory)[12]

3.11.1 HBO_2 is used in conjunction with culture-directed antibiotics and surgical debridement.

3.11.2 Chronic osteomyelitis Cierny-Mader stage 3B and 4B are considered candidates for treatment, in addition to other classifications relevant to the overlying wound such as Wagner 3 or greater in Diabetics and Tisch Classification for malignant external otitis.

3.11.3 A target oxygen level of greater or equal to 150 mmHg is recommended.

3.11.4 Treatment should be performed at 2.4-2.5 ATA for 90 minutes daily.

3.11.5 Utilization review is indicated after completion of 30-40 treatment sessions.

3.12 Delayed Radiation Injury (Soft Tissue and Bony Necrosis)[8]

3.12.1 Patients are not treated prophylactically. All patients who receive radiation therapy have subacute radiation damage manifested as obliterative endarteritis, the disease that hyperbaric oxygen treats from an evidence-based protocol.

3.12.2 Typical number of treatments are 30-60 at 2.0-2.5 ATA for 90-120 minutes depending on treatment depth.

3.12.3 Utilization review should be accomplished after 60 treatments.

3.13 Compromised Grafts and Flaps[5]

3.13.1 Treatment performed at 2.0-2.5 ATA for 90-120 minutes depending on treatment depth utilized.

3.13.2 Utilization review is required after 20 treatments when preparing a recipient site for a flap or graft.

3.13.3 Utilization review is required after 20 treatments post flap or graft has been placed into its recipient site.

3.14 Acute Thermal Burn Injury[14]

3.14.1 Hyperbaric oxygen therapy is begun as soon as possible after injury and often during initial resuscitation protocols.

3.14.2 Treatments are attempted 3 times in the first 24 hours, then twice daily beginning on Day 2.

3.14.3 Treatments are performed at 2.0-2.4 ATA for 90 minutes on 100% O_2.

3.14.4 Treatment protocols are the same for the adult and pediatric populations.

3.14.5 Utilization review is recommended after 40 hyperbaric sessions.

3.15 Idiopathic Sudden Sensorineural Hearing Loss[9]

3.15.1 Recommend 100% oxygen at 2.0-2.5 ATA for 90 minutes daily for 10-20 treatments.

3.15.2 Consider initiating HBO_2 preferably within two weeks of diagnosis but up to three months. Hyperbaric treatment and steroids should be initiated concomitantly regardless of the route of steroid treatment: intravenous infusion, intratympanic injections or oral preparations.

3.15.3 Utilization review is recommended after 20 treatments.

This is typically an emergent treatment usually in the Class A multiplace chamber setting. There are academic centers capable of managing critical patients in a Class B monoplace environment. Emergency treatment will be performed if the patient's emergency diagnosis falls within the parameters and scope of treatment specific to the institution or unit.

EMERGENCY PROCEDURES

300 HBO₂ EMERGENCY PROCEDURES

Purpose

1.1 Emergencies in the hyperbaric unit are identified and require immediate attention by the qualified and trained hyperbaric unit staff.

Policy

2.1 The hyperbaric unit staff will have initial and ongoing training for emergencies to reduce the potential for and to address emergent situations.

2.2 Every staff member has the responsibility and training to decrease the potential for fire in and around the hyperbaric chamber.

2.3 The hyperbaric physician, safety director and nurse manager are notified immediately for all emergency situations.

Procedure

A fire requires three items:

   a. An ignition source

   b. Fuel

   c. Oxygen (enough to support combustion)

3.1 Emergency Procedures:

   3.1.1 Type of emergencies

      3.1.1.1 Chamber and support equipment

      3.1.1.2 Patient care issues

3.2 The hyperbaric staff will monitor for restricted items going into the hyperbaric chamber regardless of chamber type (Class A or Class B)

   3.2.1 Every patient

   3.2.2 Every treatment

   3.2.3 Every day

3.3 The hyperbaric trained staff will have full knowledge of the oxygen shutoff valve location and when it's appropriate to discontinue supply to the chamber during fire potential. This procedure varies depending on the types of chambers utilized. Certain Class B chambers cannot be vented when the oxygen valve is closed and there's no flow. Please refer to your chamber manual for proper procedure.

3.4 Fire Drills:

3.4.1 A full-scale drill will occur every six months.

3.4.2 A review of the fire drill will occur at least quarterly.

3.4.3 At least one fire safety issue will be presented at staff meetings each month.

3.5 For fires in and/or around the chamber area:

3.5.1 Recommend job responsibility for each member of the team in conjunction with your facility procedures, for example:

3.5.1.1 Chamber operator: Turn off oxygen when appropriate (depending on types of chambers used) and remove everyone from area.

3.5.1.2 Sound alarm.

3.5.1.3 Put on alternative breathing system if needed.

3.5.1.4 Staff member: Use fire extinguisher if needed and assist with removal of people from the area.

3.5.1.5 Administrative Assistant: Call fire department; notify hospital facility.

3.5.1.6 Department director: Check rooms and put "X" on each door to signify no one is left in room.

3.5.1.7 Designate area for everyone to meet.

3.5.1.8 Document time to complete above.

3.6 Chamber and support equipment procedures to be commensurate with the types of chambers being utilized (Class A or Class B)

3.6.1 Fire

3.6.1.1 Fire in Class B monoplace chamber

3.6.1.1.1 Turn off oxygen at the chamber as soon as feasible and appropriate for type of chamber.

3.6.1.1.2 Remove everyone from the area immediately.

3.6.1.1.3 Sound alarm.

3.6.1.1.4 Take cover - recommend down close to the side of the chamber.

3.6.1.1.5 Stay away from the ends of the chamber.

3.6.1.2 Fire in Class A multiplace chamber

3.6.1.2.1 Inside observer

3.6.1.2.1.1 Notifies the chamber operator immediately

3.6.1.2.1.2 Dons built-in breathing system (BIBS) mask

3.6.1.2.1.3 Shall be certain the all patients have their hoods or BIBS masks in place

    3.6.1.2.1.4 Will use the handheld water line if fire can possibly be contained in that fashion

    3.6.1.2.1.5 Will activate the fire suppression system if the fire is deemed noncontrollable via hand line suppression

   3.6.1.2.2 Chamber operator

    3.6.1.2.2.1 Will discontinue oxygen and charge lines with air

    3.6.1.2.2.2 Will notify nearby team members for assistance

    3.6.1.2.2.3 Medical director and hyperbaric physician will be notified by available team member.

    3.6.1.2.2.4 Initiate fire alarm sequence in conjunction with the facility protocol.

    3.6.1.2.2.5 Initiate decompression of the chamber.

    3.6.1.2.2.6 Evaluate patient and inside observer decompression obligations and plan accordingly.

    3.6.1.2.2.7 Assist with safely removing everyone from the area once removed from the chamber.

3.7 Fire in the Department

 3.7.1 Class B monoplace chamber

  3.7.1.1 Turn off oxygen at the chamber and at oxygen shutoff valve at entry to chamber room when feasible, depending on chamber manufacturer guidelines and necessity for decompression.

  3.7.1.2 Put on smoke hood or alternative breathing source.

  3.7.1.3 Sound alarm.

  3.7.1.4 Contain fire, if possible.

  3.7.1.5 Evacuate patient from hyperbaric chamber when safe, being aware that oxygen will spill into room immediately as soon as the chamber door is opened and the patient's garments will be oxygen saturated.

 3.7.2 Class A multiplace chamber

  3.7.2.1 Charge treatment and BIBS gas to air.

  3.7.2.2 Notify team members for assistance.

  3.7.2.3 Sound alarm.

  3.7.2.4 Don the alternative breathing source.

  3.7.2.5 Contain fire if possible.

  3.7.2.6 Begin decompression protocols and evaluate decompression obligations of patients and inside observers.

3.7.2.7 Evacuate the chamber when safe to do so.

3.7.2.8 Abide by usual and customary missed decompression protocols, if necessary.

3.8 Fire in the Hospital (Class A and Class B chamber types)

3.8.1 Monitor situation.

3.8.2 Abort treatment if threatened.

3.8.3 Prepare to evacuate.

3.8.3.1 Action: R.A.C.E.

3.8.3.1.1 Rescue – Remove all persons in immediate danger to safety.

3.8.3.1.2 Alarm – Activate manual pull station AND have someone call 911.

3.8.3.1.3 Contain – Close doors and fire shutters to prevent spread of smoke.

3.8.3.1.4 Evacuate/Extinguish fire

3.8.3.1.4.1 Zone – Move away from immediate danger to areas within same fire zone.

3.8.3.1.4.2 Horizontal – Move to the designated evacuation zone on the same floor, usually practiced in fire drills.

3.8.3.1.4.3 Floor Evacuation – Move to a lower floor. Usually done when personnel must move to a safer level but the building is not threatened.

3.9 External Building Evacuation (completely out of building to designated emergency assembly point)

3.9.1 Chamber and support equipment

3.9.1.1 Loss of power

3.9.1.1.1 Have flashlight at chamber side – emergency lighting in place.

3.9.1.1.2 Notify patients and/or inside observers in the Class A chamber.

3.9.1.1.3 Maintain communications – limit use of chamber communication system.

3.9.1.1.4 Abort treatment (if necessary) depending on length of power failure and decompression obligations of the staff working inside the Class A chamber.

3.9.1.2 Leaks (hissing sounds)

3.9.1.2.1 Usually find during compression

3.9.1.2.2 Most common causes in a Class B chamber are linen in door or pass-through valve not tightened

3.9.1.2.3 Class A chambers can have multiple etiologies for leaks and should be evaluated by the safety director and/or the chamber manufacturer if the cause of the leak is structural.

3.9.1.2.4 Action: Decompress chamber as feasible and fix the cause.

NOTE: Do not continue to pressurize the chamber while any leaking/hissing sound is present.

3.9.1.3 Mechanical failure

    3.9.1.3.1 Abort treatment and investigate the cause of the failure.

    3.9.1.3.2 Typical problems with a Class B chamber: set pressure valve failure and door interlock switch.

    3.9.1.3.3 Possible problems with a Class A chamber: compressor failure, volume tanks losing pressure.

3.9.1.4 Loss of gas (oxygen) supply (Class B)

    3.9.1.4.1 Turn the pressure set control to zero.

    3.9.1.4.2 Turn the master selector valve to "off" position.

    3.9.1.4.3 Chamber will decompress on its own around 5 psi/minute.

    3.9.1.4.4 Notify patient.

    3.9.1.4.5 Monitor patient closely for barotrauma – remind patient to breathe regularly and not to hold breath.

    3.9.1.4.6 May open chamber door when chamber pressure indicator shows black.

3.9.1.5 Manual shutoff valve operations (Class B)

    3.9.1.5.1 There is a quick operating manual shutoff valve installed between the chamber and the pressure relief valves at the end of the chamber.

    3.9.1.5.2 The manual shutoff valve is sealed open with a frangible seal (soft wire). There is a red tag attached to each manual shutoff valve.

    3.9.1.5.3 Should a relief valve malfunction and cause rapid decompression, break the seal and close the manual shutoff valves.

3.9.1.6 Emergency vent (Class B)

    3.9.1.6.1 The emergency vent is used only in extreme emergency situations. Refer to specific manufacturer protocols.

3.9.1.7 A rapid loss of chamber pressure may result in severe injury to the patient.

    3.9.1.7.1 Lung overpressurization

    3.9.1.7.2 Embolism

    3.9.1.7.3 Barotrauma, etc.

3.10 Patient Issues (Refer to Policy Numbers 300, 301, and 302)

    3.10.1 Barotrauma on compression

        3.10.1.1 Stop compression.

        3.10.1.2 Have the patient attempt equalization with various maneuvers after stopped.

        3.10.1.3 Reduce pressure by 2 fsw if equalization impossible, being certain patient does not attempt equalization during ascent.

        3.10.1.4 Communicate with patient.

        3.10.1.5 Review clearing maneuvers.

        3.10.1.6 Resume compression once clear.

        3.10.1.7 Abort treatment if patient unable to tolerate compression after three attempts to equalize.

    3.10.2 Claustrophobia/confinement anxiety

        3.10.2.1 Talk with and console the patient.

        3.10.2.2 Decompress at a normal rate and remove the patient from the chamber.

        3.10.2.3 Educate the patient.

        3.10.2.4 Notify hyperbaric physician as a prescription for antianxiety medication may be of benefit.

        3.10.2.5 Referral of the patient to a Class A multiplace chamber may be of benefit in those patients refusing treatment in a Class B monoplace chamber.

        3.10.2.6 Referral to a Class B monoplace chamber may benefit patients refusing to wear a BIBS mask or hood.

    3.10.3 Pneumothorax on ascent

        3.10.3.1 Stop decompression.

        3.10.3.2 Notify physician.

        3.10.3.3 May elect to recompress slightly.

        3.10.3.4 Prepare for emergent chest tube placement.

        3.10.3.5 Physician may lock in to perform this procedure in a Class A chamber.

        3.10.3.6 Decompress chamber per physician order.

    3.10.4 Grand mal seizure

        3.10.4.1 Stop compression/decompression.

        3.10.4.2 Alert physician.

3.10.4.3 Keep the patient safe from injury (Class A chamber).

3.10.4.4 Wait for seizure to stop and breathing has resumed.

3.10.4.5 Based on the physician order, prepare to receive patient from the Class B monoplace chamber.

3.10.4.6 Decompress chamber at the regular rate.

3.10.4.7 Class A chamber patients may be restarted on a lower dose of oxygen ordered by the hyperbaric physician of record or hyperbaric medical director, after a 15-minute wait period and baseline mentation returns.

3.10.5 Cardiac/respiratory arrest in the Class B monoplace chamber

3.10.5.1 Stop compression/decompression.

3.10.5.2 Alert physician.

3.10.5.3 Remove patient from chamber usually in less than a minute.

3.10.5.4 Emergency button may be used.

3.10.5.5 Remove patient from chamber - begin CPR.

3.10.5.6 Remove patient from chamber side. (NOTE: Oxygen will spill out as chamber door is open.)

3.10.5.7 Remove clothing and blankets to decrease chance of spark. (NOTE: It takes the oxygen 30-40 seconds to dissipate from around the patient.)

3.10.5.8 Defibrillate after 60 seconds to decrease potential for fire.

301 PREVENTION AND MANAGEMENT OF OXYGEN TOXICITY – CNS AND PULMONARY

Purpose

1.1 Hyperbaric staff will be trained in the management of medical emergencies and complications for patients receiving hyperbaric oxygen therapy.

1.2 To decrease the potential for the incidence of oxygen toxicity

    1.2.1 Central nervous system oxygen toxicity

    1.2.2 Pulmonary oxygen toxicity

1.3 To assess the degree of oxygen toxicity and manage it promptly

Policy

2.1 The hyperbaric unit staff will be skilled in reducing the potential for and management of oxygen toxicity for the patient receiving hyperbaric oxygen treatment.

2.2 The hyperbaric physician will be notified immediately if a patient experiences signs or symptoms of oxygen toxicity during hyperbaric oxygen treatment.

Procedure

3.1 Oxygen Toxicity - Central Nervous System

    3.1.1 Risk factors include:

        3.1.1.1 Prior or current history of seizures

        3.1.1.2 Elevated body temperature

        3.1.1.3 Current therapeutic use of steroids

        3.1.1.4 History of oxygen seizures

        3.1.1.5 History of febrile seizures

        3.1.1.6 Metabolic acidosis

    3.1.2 Premonitory signs and symptoms during the hyperbaric treatment may include, but are not limited to:

        3.1.2.1 V Vision -Visual changes, blurred vision, visual hallucinations

        3.1.2.2 E Ears -Auditory hallucinations, ringing in the ears

        3.1.2.3 N Nausea - May include emesis

        3.1.2.4 T Twitching -Restlessness, numbness, focal twitching (note time, duration and site)

        3.1.2.5 I Irritability - Change in personality

        3.1.2.6 D Dizziness - Vertigo

3.1.2.7　C Convulsions - Seizure activity

3.1.6.8　C Change in mentation - Change in affect

3.1.3　Actions:

3.1.3.1　Change the source of breathing from oxygen to air (Class A and Class B when available).

3.1.3.2　Remove the patient's hood or BIBS mask (Class A).

3.1.3.3　Ask the patient to put on air mask, if possible (Class B).

3.1.3.4　Change chamber oxygen to air, if possible (Class B).

3.1.3.5　Per physician order and if patient is breathing, decrease chamber pressure and abort current hyperbaric treatment (Class B).

3.1.3.6　Remove the patient via the second lock, if available (Class A).

3.1.3.6.1　Once the seizure has resolved and patient back to baseline, wait 15 minutes and try treating with a lower oxygen dose.

3.1.3.6.2　If patient seizes a second time during an elective treatment, the hyperbaric physician may choose to abort therapy and search for secondary causes for oxygen toxicity.

3.1.3.7　Seizures occurring during prolonged treatment of Type II decompression sickness or air/gas embolism will be treated as directed by the hyperbaric physician (Class A and B).

3.2　Hypoglycemia - Central Nervous System (Grand mal seizures usually have a sudden onset. Note time and length of the seizure.)

3.2.1　Risk factors include:

3.2.1.1　Decreased blood glucose levels in patients with diabetes

3.2.1.2　Blood glucose levels may drop significantly during hyperbaric oxygen treatments.

3.2.1.2.1　Signs and symptoms of decrease in blood glucose levels during HBO_2 include are not limited to:

3.2.1.2.1.1　Diaphoresis /sweating
3.2.1.2.1.2　Thirst
3.2.1.2.1.3　Mental status change
3.2.1.2.1.4　Pale, clammy skin
3.2.1.2.1.5　Patient statement "I just don't feel right"
3.1.1.2.1.6　Patient just doesn't look right
3.1.2.2.1.7　Nausea and vomiting
3.1.2.2.1.8　Patient nonresponsive

3.2.1.3　Elevated body temperature

3.2.2 Preventive measures

3.2.2.1 Blood glucose levels for all patients will be checked by the hyperbaric staff prior to the first hyperbaric treatment. Patients with diabetes will be checked in the hyperbaric unit by the hyperbaric staff prior to every hyperbaric oxygen treatment. Patient reports of blood glucose levels taken at home or elsewhere will not be considered accurate. Refer to policy 304 for comprehensive blood glucose parameters.

3.2.2.1.1 Check with patient regarding meals and time of meals.

3.2.2.1.1.1 Provide carbohydrates and sugar during HBO_2 treatments if the following are present:

3.2.2.1.1.1.1 Blood sugar is low, less than 120 mg/dl.

3.2.2.1.1.1.2 Patient has not eaten for several hours.

3.2.2.1.1.1.3 Insulin will peak during hyperbaric treatment.

3.2.2.1.2 Know if patient is taking insulin, type, and time of administration.

3.2.2.1.3 Notify physician if patient has increased body temperature above 100.5°F for orders to decrease body temperature.

3.2.2.1.4 Use of air breaks during treatment

3.2.2.1.5 Educate patient to notify chamber operator anytime he or she feels different during the hyperbaric oxygen treatment.

3.2.3 Action

3.2.3.1 Do not change pressure in a hyperbaric chamber any time a patient is having seizure activity (TONIC phase).

3.2.3.1.1 Class B chamber - Immediately monitor and assess patient status.

3.2.3.1.2 Class A chamber - Immediately remove oxygen delivery (mask or hood).

3.2.3.2 Notify hyperbaric physician and staff immediately.

3.2.3.3 Inside attendant in the Class A chamber will notify the chamber operator.

3.2.3.4 DO NOT resume decompression during an active seizure.

3.2.3.5 Upon physician order only, return patient to surface as directed after the patient has resumed normal respirations.

3.2.3.6 Decompress chamber at regular rate.

3.2.3.7 Talk gently to patient during decompression to assist patient to reorient to surroundings.

3.2.3.7.1 Staff should be cognizant that patients can often hear you and can recall what was said to them and about them.

3.2.3.8 Note and document time of onset and approximate length of the seizure.

3.2.3.9 Follow physician orders during patient recovery period.

3.2.3.10 Check blood glucose level as soon as feasible in a Class A chamber and at completion of hyperbaric treatment in a Class B.

3.2.3.11 If indicated, check lab values.

3.2.3.12 Consider follow-up treatments at decreased pressure level.

NOTE: Oxygen toxicity seizures are self-limiting and do not predispose the patient to further oxygen-induced seizure activity in the hyperbaric environment.

Per physician order, the stable patient may be discharged home.

Per physician order, patients with symptoms may be transferred to the emergency department for follow-up.

3.3 Pulmonary Oxygen Toxicity

HBO_2 standard treatment tables decrease the potential that patients will experience pulmonary oxygen toxicity.

3.3.1 Risk factors may include, but are not limited to:

3.3.1.1 Intratracheal and bronchial irritation may develop with prolonged hyperbaric exposure.

3.3.2 Early changes are generally reversible.

3.3.3 Prolonged hyperbaric exposure may result in ARDS (Acute Respiratory Distress Syndrome).

3.3.4 Symptoms include:

3.3.4.1 Substernal irritation or burning

3.3.4.2 Tightness in the chest

3.3.4.3 Dry cough

3.3.4.4 Dyspnea on exertion

3.3.5 Notify the hyperbaric physician if signs and symptoms of pulmonary oxygen toxicity are suspected.

3.4 Pneumothorax (may occur during decompression of the hyperbaric chamber)

3.4.1 Risk Factors

3.4.1.1 Recent invasive procedures (central lines, etc.)

3.4.1.2 History of spontaneous pneumothorax (can mimic anxiety and cardiac distress)

3.4.2 A pneumothorax will get worse upon ascent.

3.4.2.1 Monitor patient and don't compress or decompress the chamber until ordered to do so by the hyperbaric physician.

3.4.3 Preventive measure: Chest auscultation prior to every HBO_2 treatment. Chest X-ray indicated for abnormal breath sounds, decreased or absent breath sounds or difficulty breathing.

3.4.4 Signs and symptoms of pneumothorax (will see on ascent)

  3.4.4.1 Sudden shortness of breath

  3.4.4.2 Sudden chest pain

  3.4.4.3 Tracheal shift toward the affected side

  3.4.4.4 Asymmetrical chest movement or lack of chest movement on affected side

  3.4.4.5 Increase in respiratory distress with decompression and relief upon recompression

3.4.5 Action

  3.4.5.1 Notify hyperbaric physician immediately.

  3.4.5.2 HOLD pressure in chamber until physician arrives and a full management team is assembled. The decision to treat a pneumothorax inside the Class A chamber may be considered in extreme circumstances such as with a tension pneumothorax and unstable vital signs. This is a hyperbaric physician decision and will be left to his or her discretion. Depending on the patient's hyperbaric diagnosis and need for hyperbaric treatment, immediate recompression (Class B chamber) or continuation of appropriate decompression schedule (Class A chamber) may be warranted at the discretion of the hyperbaric medical director or treating hyperbaric physician.

  3.4.5.3 Hyperbaric physician may choose to lock into the Class A chamber and treat the condition prior to ascent.

  3.4.5.4 Have Code/Rapid Response Team available, or

  3.4.5.5 Call 911 to have emergent responders available if located off-site of the hospital.

3.4.6 Per physician order, may elect to recompress slightly to resolve symptoms.

3.4.7 Prepare for emergent chest tube or needle placement when patient removed from the chamber by having the thoracentesis (chest tube) tray ready. (This will be performed inside Class A chamber prior to decompression.)

3.4.8 Decompress chamber per hyperbaric physician order, usually taking no more than one minute.

3.4.9 Assist in thoracentesis or insertion of chest tube or needle into the affected side (per staff qualifications).

3.4.10 Transfer patient to the Emergency Department or to 911 emergency responders.

3.4.11 Obtain STAT chest X-ray if time allows.

3.4.12 Arrange for hospital admission for outpatients.

3.4.13 Notify primary/referring/attending physician and responsible family member accompanying the patient if HIPAA compliant.

302 PREVENTION AND MANAGEMENT OF BAROTRAUMA

Purpose

1.1 Hyperbaric staff will be trained in the management of medical emergencies and complications for patients receiving hyperbaric oxygen therapy.

1.2 To decrease the potential for barotrauma by utilizing preventive measures

Policy

2.1 The hyperbaric unit staff will be skilled in reducing the potential for and management of barotrauma of ears, sinus and teeth, for the patient receiving hyperbaric oxygen treatment.

2.2 Hyperbaric staff will assess patient ears prior to and after hyperbaric treatment and document according to the TEED or O'Neill grading systems.

2.3 The hyperbaric physician will be notified immediately for patient care issues during hyperbaric oxygen treatment.

Procedure

3.1 Ear and Sinus Squeeze

    3.1.1 Risk factors include secondary causes of eustachian tube dysfunction (ETD):

        3.1.1.1 Current cold or allergy

        3.1.1.2 Ear infection

        3.1.1.3 Blocked eustachian tube

        3.1.1.4 Radiation to head/neck area

        3.1.1.5 Trauma to head/neck area

        3.1.1.6 Surgery to head/neck area

        3.1.1.7 External ear canal packing

        3.1.1.8 Endotracheal tube

3.2 Pretreatment Patient Assessment

    3.2.1 Screen patient for history of ear, sinus and tooth problems (dental caries).

    3.2.2 Screen for patient experiences with changes in pressure (flying, diving, mountain roads).

    3.2.3 Assess patient ear with attention to external auditory canal and the tympanic membrane (TM).

    3.2.4 Instruct patient on modified Valsalva maneuver and document movement of TM with equalization maneuvers.

    3.2.5 Assess tympanic membrane pre- and post-HBO$_2$ treatment, recording per TEED or O'Neill grading systems, noting level, if any, of barotrauma.

3.3 Prior to HBO$_2$ Treatment

    3.3.1 Per physician order, administer decongestant, if needed.

        3.3.1.1 Recommend nasal spray or oral decongestant based on primary or secondary ETD.

            3.3.1.1.1 Sudafed is not recommended for patients with a history of high blood pressure, prostatic hypertrophy or other potential medical conditions that may be exacerbated using this medication class.

    3.3.2 Elevate the head (semisitting or sitting) during HBO$_2$ therapy to assist in equalization of middle ear.

    3.3.3 Ensure chamber operator understands compression should stop when patient is unable to equalize ears due to pressure and should decompress until pain and/or pressure are relieved.

    3.3.4 Patient education of eustachian tube dysfunction and potential barotrauma prior to HBO$_2$ therapy:

        3.3.4.1 Methods to equalize pressure in middle ear during compression

        3.3.4.2 Patient demonstration of equalization techniques prior to every HBO$_2$ treatment

        3.3.4.3 Instruct patient to notify chamber operator immediately when pressure or fullness is felt in ear, sinus or tooth.

3.4 Changing the rate of compression of the hyperbaric chamber may allow for easier equalization of ear pressure.

    3.4.1 Monitor patient closely for any signs of pain or discomfort during compression.

3.5 Action when patient is experiencing barotrauma during pressurization:

    3.5.1 Stop compression immediately.

    3.5.2 Notify hyperbaric physician (Class B chamber) or the chamber operator (Class A chamber), who will notify the hyperbaric physician.

    3.5.3 Reduce chamber pressure until pain is resolved.

    3.5.4 Have patient perform ear clearing techniques as instructed prior to ascent.

    3.5.5 If unable to clear ears, reduce pressure further.

    3.5.6 If pain has subsided, resume compression and monitor patient closely.

    3.5.7 If pain has not resolved, abort treatment and notify physician.

    3.5.8 Assess ears when patient treatment is finished, reporting per TEED or O'Neill grading systems, noting level, if any, of barotrauma.

    3.5.9 Notify physician of patient ear, sinus or tooth pain during treatment.

    3.5.10 Future patient treatment will be held until evaluated by the hyperbaric physician.

3.5.11 An ENT consult may be required to examine and/or place PE (pressure equalizer) tubes or perform a myringotomy if needed to continue with HBO_2 treatments.

3.5.12 If patient experiences tooth squeeze, refer patient to a dentist for evaluation.

3.5.13 Patients who suffer barotrauma are not treated in the hyperbaric chamber until cleared by the hyperbaric physician.

Purpose

1.1 To decrease the potential for the incidence of confinement (claustrophobia) anxiety

1.2 To assess the degree of confinement anxiety and manage effectively

1.3 To address the psychological needs of the patient with confinement anxiety before, during, and after HBO$_2$ treatments

Policy

2.1 The patient receiving hyperbaric oxygen therapy will be evaluated for the potential for confinement anxiety to allow the staff to effectively assist the patient in managing anxiety during hyperbaric oxygen treatments.[15]

2.2 The hyperbaric physician will be notified for confinement anxiety issues prior to, during, and after hyperbaric oxygen treatment.

2.3 The staff will be skilled in the prevention and maintenance of claustrophobia/confinement anxiety.

Procedure

3.1 Notify hyperbaric physician immediately for signs of confinement anxiety. Confinement anxiety/claustrophobia can occur before the treatment, or at any time during any HBO$_2$ treatment. Confinement anxiety may be a single or intermittent occurrence, or may be an ongoing chronic problem.

    3.1.1 Assess the patient for degree of confinement anxiety.[15]

        3.1.1.1 Patients may admit to having claustrophobia/confinement anxiety.

        3.1.1.2 Assess patient's fear of closed spaces. (A history of prior response to being enclosed in an MRI scanner may be helpful.)

    3.1.2 Orient patient to hyperbaric oxygen therapy.[15]

        3.1.2.1 Emphasize systematic patient orientation desensitization process by:

            3.1.2.1.1 Familiarizing patient with chamber unit

            3.1.2.1.2 Letting patient observe other patients receiving HBO$_2$ therapy (with verbal consent from patients being treated)

            3.1.2.1.3 Having patient lie down on HBO$_2$ stationary gurney (Class B chamber) or sit in the chamber seat (Class A chamber)

            3.1.2.1.4 Staying with patient for constant psychological support as patient adjusts to environment

            3.1.2.1.5 Pushing gurney halfway into chamber, allowing patient to express feelings of anxiety (Class B chamber)

            3.1.2.1.6 Asking patient if he/she is ready to proceed farther into the chamber. If not, wait until willing to proceed. If still not ready, reschedule treatment, try again, or per physician order, offer to provide anti-anxiety medication

        3.1.2.1.7 Administer medication as prescribed by HBO_2 physician.

            3.1.2.1.7.1 Recommend oral anti-anxiety medication be given at least 45 minutes prior to HBO_2 treatment.

    3.1.2.2 Use appropriate relaxation techniques and/or diversional activities while patient is in the chamber.

        3.1.2.2.1 Have patient watch TV.

        3.1.2.2.2 Hyperbaric nurse, technician, and family member to sit by chamber to reduce patient anxiety

        3.1.2.2.3 The physician may choose to lock into the Class A chamber to provide psychological support to the patient.

3.1.3 Monitor the patient for signs and symptoms of confinement anxiety:

    3.1.3.1 Hyperventilation

    3.1.3.2 Clenching of fists

    3.1.3.3 Sudden complaint of discomfort

    3.1.3.4 Urgency to empty the bladder

    3.1.3.5 Feelings of being smothered or suffocated

    3.1.3.6 Flushed face

    3.1.3.7 Profuse diaphoresis

3.1.4 Monitor patient for subtle signs of anxiety reaction. Handle situation with sensitivity.

    3.1.4.1 Defensive attitude

    3.1.4.2 Flat affect

3.1.5 Intervene in a sudden claustrophobic anxiety reaction.

    3.1.5.1 Let patient know you are beginning to decompress chamber and that it will take time.

    3.1.5.2 Patient may also be offered to lock out through the emergency/transfer lock in a Class A multiplace chamber without interruption of other patient's treatment.

    3.1.5.3 Coach patient to breathe slowly using his or her abdominal muscles.

    3.1.5.4 Stay with the patient and maintain communication (verbal and audio) at all times.

    3.1.5.5 Direct the patient to perform some distracting tasks such as counting, reciting his/her address and telephone number.

3.1.5.6 Inform the patient of approximate time treatment will end.

3.1.6 When chamber is at surface, open door and remove the patient.

3.1.6.1 Offer support and understanding to patient's reaction.

3.1.6.1.1 Talk to the patient, encourage the patient to discuss feelings.

3.1.7 Transport patient back to room or discharge home if patient calm.

304 BLOOD GLUCOSE PARAMETERS

Purpose

1.1 To reduce the potential for hypoglycemic reaction during hyperbaric oxygen treatments for patients with diabetes

1.2 Hypoglycemic reaction may precipitate oxygen toxic seizure activity.

Policy

2.1 Patients with diabetes will have blood glucose levels checked by the hyperbaric staff prior to and after each hyperbaric treatment.

Procedure

3.1 Determine and document the type of medication (oral, insulin or both), dose and time patient takes the medication.

3.2 Determine and document the peak time for insulin.

3.3 Determine and document time of patient meal and what he or she ate.

3.4 Check blood glucose level with glucometer as per usual protocol.

3.5 Patients with a diagnosis of diabetes that are:

    3.5.1 Non-insulin dependent (diet-controlled/do not take medication for diabetes)

        3.5.1.1 Check blood glucose level prior to HBO_2 treatment.

        3.5.1.2 If blood glucose is greater than 90 mg/dL, begin HBO_2 treatment.

        3.5.1.3 If blood glucose level is less than 90 mg/dL, give glucose/carbohydrate/protein supplementation.

        3.5.1.4 Recheck blood glucose level in 15 minutes.

        3.5.1.5 If blood glucose level is over 90, may begin HBO_2 treatment. If under 90, notify hyperbaric physician for further orders.

    3.5.2 Non-insulin dependent (oral medication for diabetes)

        3.5.2.1 Check blood glucose level prior to HBO_2 treatment.

        3.5.2.2 If blood glucose level is greater than 100 mg/dL, begin HBO_2 treatment.

        3.5.2.3 If blood glucose level is less than 100 mg/dL, give glucose/carbohydrate/protein supplementation.

        3.5.2.4 Recheck blood glucose level in 15 minutes.

        3.5.2.5 If blood glucose level is over 100, may begin HBO_2 treatment. If under 100, notify hyperbaric physician for further orders.

3.5.3 Insulin dependent (takes insulin)

    3.5.3.1 Check blood glucose prior to HBO_2 treatment.

    3.5.3.2 If blood glucose level greater than 120 mg/dL, may begin HBO_2 treatment.

    3.5.3.3 If blood glucose level is less than 120 mg/dL, give glucose/carbohydrate/protein supplementation. Note time, amount and type of last insulin dose. Note when and what patient last ate.

    3.5.3.4 Recheck blood glucose level in 15 minutes and if over 120 mg/dL, may begin HBO_2 treatment. If under 120 mg/dL, notify hyperbaric physician for further orders and glucose/carbohydrate/protein supplementation (IV or oral).

3.6 Instruct patient to notify the hyperbaric chamber operator if he or she is experiencing any changes related to hypoglycemia during the HBO_2 treatment. Symptoms vary among patients so they may know best when this is occurring.

3.7 Check blood glucose levels on all patients with diabetes post hyperbaric treatment. Notify the hyperbaric physician if any changes in blood glucose levels.

Purpose

1.1 To ensure safety related to absolute and relative medical contraindications to treatment as with hyperbaric oxygen treatment

1.2 The hyperbaric center staff will be responsible for understanding and promoting a safe environment in the hyperbaric department.

Policy

2.1 The hyperbaric center staff will be familiar with medications that are determined to have absolute and/or relative contraindications for use by patients receiving hyperbaric oxygen treatments.

Procedure

3.1 Absolute Contraindication:

    3.1.1 Untreated pneumothorax

3.2 Relative Contraindications:

    3.2.1 Asthma

    3.2.2 Congenital spherocytosis

    3.2.3 Emphysema with CO_2 retention

    3.2.4 High fever

    3.2.5 History of optic neuritis

    3.2.6 History of otosclerosis surgery

    3.2.7 History of spontaneous pneumothorax

    3.2.8 History of thoracic surgery

    3.2.9 Implanted medical devices such as but not limited to, a pacemaker, defibrillator, ventriculoperitoneal shunt, penile implant, medication ports (check with manufacturer for pressure rating)

    3.2.10 Pregnancy

    3.2.11 Seizure disorders

    3.2.12 Upper respiratory infection and chronic sinusitis

    3.2.13 Viral infections

3.3 Use the following guidelines for patients who may be taking or have recently taken the following medications. Treatment of patients who may be using these medications must be approved by the medical director.

3.3.1 Antabuse - Predisposes to oxygen toxicity

3.3.2 Antiseizure medications - Check therapeutic levels. Low levels can predispose to oxygen toxicity.

3.3.3 Meclizine - Predisposes to oxygen toxicity

3.3.4 Bleomycin

    3.3.4.1 May cause pulmonary fibrosis that can lead to air embolism or pneumothorax in the patient receiving hyperbaric oxygen treatment.

3.3.5 Certain ointments/creams that cannot be removed, may be covered with cotton dressings.

3.3.6 Narcotics - Can lead to cessation of the hypoxic respiratory drive.

3.3.7 Nitroprusside – HBO_2 vasoconstrictive effect interacts with nitroprusside's vasodilator effect, making intensive monitoring mandatory.

3.3.8 Penicillin - Predisposes to oxygen toxicity

3.3.9 Promethazine (Phenergan) - Predisposes to oxygen toxicity. Switch to another anti-emetic.

3.3.10 Steroids - Decreases the threshold for oxygen toxicity.

3.3.11 Sulfamylon - Promotes CO_2 buildup causing peripheral vasodilatation. When coupled with vasoconstriction, results are worse than with using either agent alone. Use silver sulfadiazine instead.

3.3.12 Vitamin A, in excess, may retard healing.

3.3.13 Vitamin E - Normal doses of Vitamin E (800 IU QD) reduce free radicals.

306 BOMB THREAT

Purpose

1.1 Hyperbaric staff will be prepared to respond to a bomb threat received by the hyperbaric center.

Policy

2.1 Hyperbaric staff will safely and quickly remove all personnel and patients to a safe location outside of the wound healing and hyperbaric center to a predetermined location.

2.2 Regardless of outcome, it is best to consider all such threats as substantial until proven otherwise.

Procedure

3.1 In the event of a bomb threat:

    3.1.1 The staff shall quickly and safely evacuate all persons from the hyperbaric center to a safe location.

    3.1.2 The department director shall take a head count of all persons in the center before and after evacuation.

    3.1.3 The hyperbaric department director or acting senior nurse or technician shall call in threat to 911 Emergency.

3.2 If a hyperbaric treatment is underway within the department, prompt and safe termination of the treatment shall be conducted per the following guidelines. The chamber personnel shall perform the following based on the type of chamber:

    3.2.1 Monoplace chamber procedures (Class B chamber)

        3.2.1.1 Decompress the patients at a normal travel rate.

        3.2.1.2 If danger is imminent, the decompression rate may be increased to the maximum travel rate of 60 fpm (1 ft/sec).

        3.2.1.3 Calm and reassure all patients.

        3.2.1.4 Remove the patient(s) from the chamber and prepare for transport to the safe area.

        3.2.1.5 Shut down system as applicable and assist with patient transport and support as required.

        3.2.1.6 Turn off and unplug all electrical equipment.

        3.2.1.7 Shut down system as necessary for safe departure.

    3.2.2 Multiplace chamber procedures (Class A chamber)

        3.2.2.1 Inside observer:

            3.2.2.1.1 If it will affect therapy, inform the patients of the situation.

3.2.2.1.2 Ensure patients that the chamber is one of the safest places in the area.

3.2.2.1.3 Prepare to abort treatment if necessary.

3.2.2.1.4 Remove the patient(s) from the chamber and prepare for transport.

3.2.2.2 Chamber operator:

3.2.2.2.1 Inform medical director and safety director.

3.2.2.2.2 Have decompression profile and treatment termination procedure prepared.

3.2.2.2.3 Decompress the patients at a normal travel rate.

3.2.2.2.4 If danger is imminent, then decompression rate may be increased to the maximum travel rate of 1 foot every two seconds (30 fpm).

3.2.2.2.5 Remove the patient(s) from the chamber and prepare for transport.

3.2.2.2.6 Shut down system as applicable and assist with patient transport and support as required.

3.2.2.2.7 Turn off and unplug all electrical equipment.

3.2.2.2.8 Shut down system as necessary for safe departure.

3.2.2.2.9 If any inside observer has skipped a decompression, place on 100% oxygen and notify the hyperbaric physician.

3.3 Other Staff: Threats by Mail

3.3.1 Be alert for suspicious-looking letters/packages.

3.3.2 If you are suspicious of a package, DO NOT HANDLE IT.

3.3.3 Notify Security at 911.

3.4 Threats by Telephone

3.4.1 Notify Security at 911.

3.4.2 Follow Bomb Threat Checklist to record as many details as possible.

3.4.3 Return to your work area and begin visual inspection.

3.4.4 DO NOT TOUCH ANY SUSPICIOUS OBJECTS OR PACKAGES.

3.4.5 Report any suspicious objects or packages to Security 911.

3.4.6 Follow any instructions from building manager/administrator.

3.4.7 Prepare to evacuate to assembly area if object found.

3.5 Safety Director:

3.5.1 Coordinate information flow and treatment termination procedure.

3.5.2 Oversee decompression and patient/staff safety responsibilities.

3.5.3 Limit phone calls to emergencies.

3.5.4 Do not allow use of cell phones.

3.5.5 Prepare to assist with dive termination procedure and evacuation if needed.

3.6 Medical Director

3.6.1 Prepare to terminate hyperbaric oxygen therapy if necessary.

3.6.2 Make the ultimate decision to terminate patient treatment.

3.6.3 Be prepared for the need to handle missed decompression of inside observers.

307 PATIENT RESTRAINTS DURING HYPERBARIC TREATMENTS

Purpose

1.1   To prevent injury while providing a safe environment for patients requiring restraint during HBO_2 treatment

Policy

2.1   Patients with altered levels of consciousness may require the use of restraints to prevent injury.

Procedure

3.1   Equipment Needed

   3.1.1   Soft limb restraints without Velcro

   3.1.2   Cotton sheet for chest restraint, if needed

3.2   Procedure

   3.2.1   Determine level of consciousness of the patient to determine if restraints are needed to prevent the patient from causing harm while receiving HBO_2 treatments.

   3.2.2   Restraints are used per hyperbaric physician order and hospital policy.

   3.2.3   Soft limb restraints are used at the wrist and ankles as needed and tied under the HBO_2 gurney away from the rollers and under the mattress.

   3.2.4   The patient's hands may need to be wrapped with the soft restraint (without Velcro) to keep the patient from pulling at equipment.

   3.2.5   It may be necessary to tie a cotton sheet around the patient's chest and/or legs to keep the patient from lifting the upper torso or legs. Tie the sheets under the mattress.

   3.2.6   Keep the hands and feet visible to monitor the restraints for proper placement.

   3.2.7   Document the condition of the hands and feet every 15 minutes to ensure the restraints remain in place and there are no signs of the restraints being too tight.

   3.2.8   Consider referral to a Class A multiplace chamber if treatment in the Class B monoplace chamber is not feasible.

308 CELL PHONE AND OTHER PERSONAL ELECTRONIC DEVICES

Purpose

1.1 To avoid distraction by the hyperbaric chamber operator during hyperbaric oxygen treatment

1.2 To avoid cell phones and other personal electronic devices being taken into the hyperbaric chamber by staff and patients

Policy

2.1 Chamber operator(s) are not allowed to use cell phones and other personal electronic devices for nonessential activity/purpose during chamber(s) operations.

2.2 Chamber operations are defined as patient treatment, chamber maintenance, chamber cleaning, and chamber pressurization for any reason.

2.3 Nonessential is defined as any activity/purpose that does not involve direct care and oversight for the patient receiving hyperbaric oxygen treatment.

Procedure

3.1 It is the responsibility of the chamber operator to remain alert to the condition of the chamber(s) and occupant(s).

3.2 Hyperbaric chamber operator's cell phone and/or other electronic devices are to be stored in/on a space away from the hyperbaric chamber during:

    3.2.1 Preparation for hyperbaric chamber treatment

    3.2.2 Patient receiving hyperbaric oxygen treatment

    3.2.3 Cleaning of the hyperbaric chamber

    3.2.4 Maintenance of hyperbaric chamber

    3.2.5 Pressurization of the hyperbaric chamber for any reason

3.3 Patients will be screened for the presence of cell phones or electronic devices prior to each hyperbaric oxygen treatment.

3.4 Hyperbaric staff will check to ensure cell phones and/or other personal electronic devices are stored in/on a space away from the chamber during the events listed in 3.2 above.

3.5 Violation of the use of cell phones and other personal electronic devices per this policy may result in immediate dismissal.

PATIENT CARE

400 PATIENT ADMISSION SCREENING

Purpose

1.1 The office coordinator, and where appropriate, the intake/DME coordinator will collect patient information to ensure proper identification for scheduling, assignment to practitioners and billing.

Policy

2.1 The hyperbaric physician of record shall medically screen every new patient for appropriateness of admission to the program and refer to the hyperbaric director or nurse manager for appropriate orientation to the department.

2.2 Patient information is required to assure appropriate services will be managed by hyperbaric center.

2.3 Preauthorization for hyperbaric oxygen therapy will be submitted as necessary per CMS and private insurance guidelines.

Procedure

3.1 The hyperbaric physicians will determine if a patient is a candidate for hyperbaric oxygen therapy utilizing established criteria.

3.2 Initiate and complete patient preregistration form. The information includes, but is not limited to:

    3.2.1 Patient information section: name, SSN, address, phone number, date of birth, age, race, sex and marital status

    3.2.2 Guarantor name, address and phone number

    3.2.3 Employment information

    3.2.4 Pharmacy and phone number

3.3 Referral Information Section

    3.3.1 List referral source

    3.3.2 Attending, referring, and family physician (include phone numbers)

    3.3.3 State how patient heard about center

3.4 Insurance Information:

    3.4.1 Insurance company name

    3.4.2 Policy/referral numbers

    3.4.3 Precertification if needed

    3.4.4 Copy front and back of insurance cards; ensure legibility.

    3.4.5 Document who verified insurance.

3.5 Schedule patient with the hyperbaric physician requested by the patient or patient's family or the on-call hyperbaric physician when the patient is referred directly to the hyperbaric department.

3.6 Instruct patient to bring the following:

    3.6.1 Insurance cards

    3.6.2 List of current medications

    3.6.3 Any recent medical records (reports, etc.)

    3.6.4 List of transportation sources for the patient verbally or in writing

3.7 All patients shall be registered/admitted according to the hospital's admission procedures including assignment of a medical record number.

3.8 The office secretary shall investigate insurance coverage. Indicate on the registration form the patient's insurance benefits. Copy both sides of all insurance cards.

3.9 The insurance company shall be contacted to verify insurance coverage using information obtained from patient intake form and copies of insurance cards. The insurance verification form shall be utilized to document this information.

3.10 Insurance verification is completed as soon as possible prior to the patient's initial visit.

3.11 The following, when appropriate, shall also occur:

    3.11.1 Worker's compensation is verified prior to first visit to obtain verification of coverage and claim number.

    3.11.2 Medicaid is verified.

    3.11.3 Managed Care Programs require authorization prior to any visits.

        3.11.3.1 An authorization number and signature must be received at the bottom of the form before the patient can be seen.

        3.11.3.2 Only the services authorized can be provided.

3.12 Any insurance that requires preauthorization is verified prior to the first visit.

3.13 Insurance cards are copied for distribution (one each) as follows:

    3.13.1 Business office

    3.13.2 Hyperbaric physician's office (if the patient has not yet been evaluated for hyperbaric oxygen therapy)

    3.13.3 Patient's medical record

    3.13.4 DME coordinator

3.14 Any problems or issues identified through verification are submitted to the department director immediately.

3.14.1 In the event an individual payment plan needs to be developed (private pay), the business office personnel shall advise and develop the plan with the patient and/or person responsible for payment.

3.14.2 Insurance verification forms and copies of insurance cards are filed in the consents/registration information section of the patient record.

3.14.3 The patient may be processed as a new or a recurring patient.

3.15 The Patient Intake Form shall be forwarded to the secretary/receptionist for chart preparation and assembly of a file folder to be forwarded to the business office within three working days. The folder shall include the following:

3.15.1 Face sheet with diagnosis

3.15.2 Insurance cards

3.15.3 Notes indicating payment arrangements

3.15.4 If applicable, notice of non-covered/coverage

3.15.5 Limitation (Medicaid only)

3.16 During the admission process, the patient's signature and/or informed consent may be obtained on the following:

3.16.1 Admission Sheet

3.16.2 Consent to Treatment and Admission - This is explained to the patient before signing. The original copy is filed in the patient's chart; a duplicate copy is given to the patient.

3.16.3 Authorization for Release of Information

3.16.4 Patient Insurance Profile - One copy is given to the patient; the second copy is filed in the patient's chart. The Billing Information Sheet explains the billing process at the hyperbaric center.

3.17 All procedures performed shall be entered into the hospital computer using the patient's medical record number (or hospital-specific protocol) to maintain accurate records of the department's activity, expenses and revenues.

3.18 Patients will be notified of amount of co-pay or out-of-pocket expense prior to treatment.

401 PATIENT INFORMED CONSENT

Purpose

1.1   The purpose of informed consent is to inform the patient of expected outcomes, benefits, and risks that may occur during his or her treatment regime.

1.2   It provides a basis for open communication between the patient (may include patient's family/significant other/patient representative) and physician to allow the patient to be an active participant in determining his or her treatment plan, care, and services.

Policy

2.1   Patient Informed Consents will be obtained for

    2.1.1   Hyperbaric oxygen therapy (including risks - oxygen toxicity, barotrauma, pneumothorax, fire)

    2.1.2   Photography

    2.1.3   General wound care treatment (for those centers that incorporate wound care into their program)

    2.1.4   Debridement or other invasive procedures

    2.1.5   Additional or special procedures

Procedure

3.1   Consents will be provided by the hospital and include at a minimum, consents for treatment, hyperbaric oxygen therapy, photography and procedures, as applicable.

3.2   Patients will be informed of the likelihood of achieving goals, reasonable alternatives, relevant risks benefits and side effects related to alternatives, including the possible results of not receiving care, treatment and services.

3.3   If the patient is a minor or unable to give informed consent, a duly authorized patient representative may sign the informed consent form.

3.4   Patient Informed Consent for hyperbaric oxygen therapy will be obtained for each course of treatment with the number of treatments expected clearly delineated. Any deviation over this number will require the signing of an additional consent for those treatments.

3.5   A copy of the original signed consent placed in the patient record according to hospital policy will be provided to patient or patient representative upon request.

402 PATIENT ORIENTATION AND TEACHING

Purpose

1.1 To prepare the patient, family and/or significant other(s) physically and emotionally for HBO_2 treatments[15]

1.2 To clearly define safety measures and outline all effects of HBO_2

1.3 To familiarize patients with techniques of air clearance (middle-ear equalization of pressure)

Policy

2.1 Patients and/or family will receive patient orientation and education with respect to HBO_2 therapy.

2.2 Teaching will be reinforced as indicated.

Procedure

3.1 Assess patient's knowledge and readiness for HBO_2.

    3.1.1 Ask patient what he/she knows about HBO_2.

    3.1.2 Ascertain what physician has communicated with the patient regarding HBO_2.

    3.1.3 Give patient an information brochure to read.

3.2 Familiarize the patient with the purposes, effects and the procedures of HBO_2 and safety precautions used.

    3.2.1 Explain the benefit of HBO_2 to the patient's specific condition.

    3.2.2 Discuss possible side effects and risks.

    3.2.3 Emphasize safety precautions to be taken and the reversibility of side effects.

    3.2.4 Restricted items include but are not limited to:

        3.2.4.1 No makeup, oils or hair spray allowed in the chamber

        3.2.4.2 No battery-operated equipment

        3.2.4.3 100% cotton or a cotton/polyester blend of at least 50% cotton garments only allowed inside chamber

        3.2.4.4 No fire fuel objects such as paper in chamber

3.3 Familiarize patients to the chamber, HBO_2 unit and personnel, and appropriate policies and procedures.

    3.3.1 Show the chamber unit and the different features for communication and diversion activity present.

    3.3.2 If patient is in his/her room, show pictures of the chamber.

    3.3.3 Discuss visiting requirements and restrictions.

3.3.4 Have hyperbaric-specific informed consent signed, dated and timed.

3.4 Instruct patients on what specific medications to take and not to take while having HBO_2 treatment as an outpatient. Coordinate care with in-house staff when inpatient.

3.4.1 Screen present medications.

3.4.2 Notify the hyperbaric physician if medications being taken are potentially contraindicated during hyperbaric oxygen treatment.

3.4.3 Coordinate with the nurse taking care of the patient regarding administration of certain drugs (e.g. insulin) and the hyperbaric oxygen treatment schedule.

3.5 Reinforce no-smoking rule.

3.6 Demonstrate auto-inflationary techniques to equalize ear pressure and encourage return demonstration.

3.6.1 Teach patient Valsalva maneuver prior to treatment and test for effectiveness.

3.7 If air breaks are given, have patient practice using mask prior to the first treatment in a Class B monoplace chamber.

3.8 Offer emotional support through a systematic desensitization process to the chamber and/or systematic technique.

403 HYPERBARIC OXYGEN TREATMENT

Purpose

1.1 To safely administer hyperbaric oxygen treatments (HBO_2) to patient in either a Class B monoplace or Class A multiplace hyperbaric chamber

1.2 To communicate to other health team members the patient's response to the HBO_2 treatment and any complications

Policy

2.1 The safe and effective preparation of the patient and the hyperbaric chamber are established for the patient receiving HBO_2 treatments.

Procedure

3.1 Equipment needed

   3.1.1 Hyperbaric chamber

   3.1.2 HBO_2 chamber cart (stretcher specifically mated to the railing system)(Class B)

   3.1.3 Oxygen supply inlet properly connected to the chamber and exhaust in accordance with proper NFPA (National Fire Protection Agency) code (Class B).

   3.1.4 Hyperbaric chamber, operations console, oxygen breathing source for all patients and inside observers in the Class A multiplace chamber (tubing, hoods and BIBS masks).

3.2 Preparation of the hyperbaric chamber for HBO_2 treatment

   3.2.1 Perform a general visual inspection of the HBO_2 chamber for damage inside and out, loose connections, crazing of acrylics, etc.

   3.2.2 Perform pretreatment chamber checklists specific for the type of chamber (Class A or Class B) daily prior to starting HBO_2 treatments.

   3.2.3 Perform patient pretreatment checklists prior to each hyperbaric treatment specific for chamber type Class A or Class B.

   3.2.4 Turn on main oxygen valve at wall and verify that the oxygen supply pressure is between 50 and 70 psig (for Class B chambers rated to 3 ATA) and minimally 120 psig for Class A chambers rated to 6 ATA.

   3.2.5 The oxygen flow meter to the chamber (Class B) or to the patient's hood or BIBS mask is set at the minimum flow rate for the chamber model used and/or adjusted for patient comfort, proper flow through the hood or BIBS mask.

3.3 Prepare the patient for the HBO_2 treatment

   3.3.1 Follow-up on initial patient orientation for any questions, concerns, problems, etc.

   3.3.2 Check to be sure the hyperbaric treatment consent is signed.

3.3.3 Perform patient pretreatment checklist prior to starting every treatment, including safety time-out/pause STOP. (Refer to Policy Guideline 408.)

3.3.4 Place patient on special cart provided for HBO_2 chamber having head at distal end of cart from the chamber (Class B monoplace) or sit the patient comfortably (Class A multiplace) or place patient on the hyperbaric-approved stretcher (Class A multiplace).

3.3.5 Use either 100% cotton linens or a blend of cotton-polyester (at least 50% cotton) for patients inside the HBO_2 chamber.

3.3.6 Visually inspect the patient for adherence to the safety protocol as outlined in "Prevention of Fire during HBO_2," procedure and remove any restricted materials or correct any deficiencies.

3.3.7 Ground the patient using the chamber ground wire attached to the cart (Class B monoplace).

3.3.8 Check the ground wire prior to every hyperbaric treatment (Class B monoplace).

3.3.9 Ensure that there is an oxygen hood or BIBS mask for each patient and inside observer (Class A).

3.3.10 Ensure that all patients have neck rings donned for entry into the multiplace chamber if hoods are utilized (Class A).

3.3.11 Ensure that all tubing is connected to the patients neck rings (Class A).

3.3.12 Ensure neck ring rubber damns are properly fitted, secure and not damaged (rips or tears) (Class A).

3.3.13 Assess the need for physiological monitoring.

3.3.14 Follow-up assessment of patient's psychological status.

3.3.15 Do not have fluorescent lights on over chamber when patient is being treated (Class B monoplace), as they may precipitate seizure activity.

3.4 Follow HBO_2 treatment operational sequence

3.4.1 Roll transfer cart into position where cart pins interlocks with chamber track sockets and lock cart wheels (Class B). Assist patients into the chamber to be seated (Class A).

3.4.2 Roll cart into chamber and allow stretcher latch to engage. Unlock transfer cart wheels and roll dolly away from chamber (Class B).

3.4.3 Gently close and lock chamber door of the Class B monoplace chamber. Establish communications system is working and the close main lock door to the Class A multiplace chamber.

3.4.4 Turn on/off selector to the "on" position immediately (Class B).

3.4.5 Complete pretreatment checklist between chamber operator and inside observer (Class A).

3.4.6 Set pressure rate controls at a comfortable rate to help the patient equalize the middle ears (Class A and Class B).

3.4.6.1 Start at 1 psig and increase to 1½ to 2 psig/minute if patient tolerates. (Generally a minimum of 10 minutes should be employed for compression to treatment depth.)

3.4.6.2 Monitor closely for eustachian tube dysfunction and possible ear barotrauma.

3.4.7 Set pressure control gauge to the treatment pressure ordered by the physician, in increments as tolerated by the patient (Class B).

3.4.8 Compress the Class A chamber at predetermined descent rate as ordered by the physician and tolerated by the patients and inside observers (Class A).

3.4.9 Set timer for 90 minutes for treatments without air breaks or as required to appropriately time air breaks as ordered (Class B).

3.4.10 Set timers accordingly for 90 minutes of oxygen breathing separated by air breaks as ordered by the hyperbaric physician (Class A).

3.4.11 When treatment time is completed, adjust pressure control to zero (Class B). Unless otherwise ordered by physician, decompress at rate compressed.

3.4.12 When treatment is completed, the chamber operator will notify the inside observer to discontinue oxygen breathing, remove hoods or masks, prepare the chamber for ascent and notify chamber operator when everyone is ready to decompress (Class A).

3.4.13 The chamber operator will charge the lines to air prior to decompression if oxygen decompression by inside observers is not needed (Class A).

3.4.14 The chamber operator will notify the inside observer that decompression will begin (Class A).

3.4.15 The inside observer will in turn notify the patients and be certain all patients are awake for ascent (Class A).

3.4.16 Decompression rate will be set as ordered by the hyperbaric physician with or without inside observer oxygen breathing.

3.4.17 Turn the on/off selector to the "off" position when chamber pressure gauge reaches 2 psig or less (Class B).

3.4.18 Open chamber door gently when chamber pressure indicators show all black (Class B).

3.4.19 Open chamber door when chamber at surface (Class A).

3.4.20 Connect and lock transfer cart to chamber, release stretcher lock-pin and roll stretcher on to cart until latch engages (Class B).

3.4.21 Chamber is to be prepared for the next treatment.

3.5 Documentation of HBO$_2$ treatment

3.5.1 Log the treatment time in the appropriate log. Indicate date, treatment number, ATA, length of treatment and any pertinent comments.

3.5.2 Class A chamber inside observers total time of dive (TTD) will also be recorded.

3.5.3 Chart treatment on Hyperbaric Treatment Record.

3.5.4 Document response and any complications or adverse effects.

3.5.5 Physician documentation of attendance with physician signature

404 HYPERBARIC TREATMENT DOCUMENTATION

Purpose

1.1 Documentation will be recorded for the chamber, treatment and patient information.

Policy

2.1 Patient hyperbaric oxygen treatment will be documented fully with all technical information and patient response to treatment.

Procedure

3.1 Record the required information (see sample form in appendices) as well as any other events or responses that might occur prior to, during or immediately after HBO_2 treatment.

405 AIR BREAKS DURING HBO₂ TREATMENT

Purpose

1.1 Air breaks are recommended for patients receiving hyperbaric oxygen treatments that are 90 minutes or longer.

1.2 Treatment and air breaks will be based upon the medical decision of the hyperbaric physician and may be modified according to the medical condition of the patient or patients being treated.

Policy

2.1 Air breaks will be ordered by the treating hyperbaric physician to decrease the potential for oxygen toxicity during hyperbaric oxygen treatment.

Procedure

3.1 Air Break Guidelines:

    3.1.1 For ensuring the highest levels of compliance, the minimal recommended air-break protocol is to give a 5-to-10-minute air break after each 20-30 minutes of 100% oxygen breathing while under pressure (2.0-3.0 ATA).

    3.1.2 Air breaks may be eliminated or modified depending on treatment times and depths, as ordered by the hyperbaric physician.

3.2. Instruct and have patient demonstrate how to use the mask for air breaks prior to hyperbaric treatment in the Class B monoplace chamber.

3.3 Air breaks in the Class A multiplace chamber can be accomplished by removing the patient's oxygen hood or mask or changing the breathing gas to air.

406 PATIENT ASSESSMENT

Purpose

1.1 To ensure that every patient is adequately assessed by hyperbaric trained personnel prior to receiving hyperbaric oxygen (HBO_2) treatment

Policy

2.1 Patient shall be evaluated and cleared for treatment prior to each hyperbaric oxygen treatment by designated personnel according to the following procedures.

Procedure

3.1 Patients that are to receive hyperbaric oxygen therapy will be screened, evaluated and approved for treatment by a physician trained and credentialed in hyperbaric medicine and with the appropriate experience commensurate with the types of chambers to be utilized (Class A, Class B or both).

3.2 Patients that are to receive hyperbaric oxygen therapy are to be evaluated by a trained hyperbaric registered nurse.

    3.2.1 The registered nurse will initiate a patient-specific nursing plan of care following the Baromedical Nurses Association (BNA) recommended guidelines.[15]

3.3 The registered hyperbaric nurse ensures the following documentation is in the medical record prior to the patient receiving HBO_2.

    3.3.1 Hyperbaric treatment order by physician trained and credentialed in hyperbaric medicine and with the appropriate experience commensurate with the types of chambers being utilized (Class A, Class B or both)

    3.3.2 Hyperbaric-specific informed consent signed by the physician and the patient

    3.3.3 Patient-specific hyperbaric plan of care

    3.3.4 Hyperbaric-specific patient education

    3.3.5 Pretreatment assessment of patients (and inside attendants in a Class A chamber), including appropriate exams/procedures that may include a chest X-ray, pulmonary function studies, pressure equalization tubes, transcutaneous oxygen monitoring, etc. with copies of all exams on the patient's chart prior to initiating treatment

    3.3.6 Patients have received any/all medications prior, during and post treatment and that medication data is recorded in each patient's chart.

    3.3.7 Patients with diabetes receive adequate caloric intake to reduce the potential for hypoglycemia during the hyperbaric treatment. (Refer to Policy Guideline 304.)

    3.3.8 The hyperbaric technologist is responsible to do the following:

        3.3.8.1 Report any irregular event(s) that occur during the hyperbaric treatment.

        3.3.8.2 Report the event(s) to the hyperbaric physician and/or chamber operator (Class A).

3.3.8.3 Post treatment blood glucose levels are checked for patients with diabetes. (Refer to Policy Guideline 304.)

    3.2.8.3.1 Abnormal results (> 350 mm/dl or < 60 mg/dl) are reported to the hyperbaric physician.

3.3.8.4 Ensure all intratreatment events and patient response to treatment are documented in the patient chart.

3.3.8.5 Keep open line of communication with the hyperbaric physician to report any adverse reactions or irregularities found during hyperbaric oxygen treatment.

3.4 Prehyperbaric oxygen therapy assessment will be performed and documented prior to EVERY HBO$_2$ treatment, to include, but not limited to:

3.4.1 Vital signs - temperature, pulse, respirations, blood pressure and pain assessment

    3.4.1.1 Patients with temperatures of 99.8°F or higher shall be evaluated by the hyperbaric physician and treated appropriately before the patient is placed in the hyperbaric chamber.

3.4.2 Ear canals, tympanic membranes and/or PE tubes visually examined for obstructions and/or presence of injury/damage.

3.4.3 Fire Safety Checklist

3.4.4 Lung auscultated for character of breath sounds

3.4.5 Indwelling tubes such as intravenous catheters, Heplock, drains, Foley catheters, etc. should be properly vented during treatment.

3.4.6 Blood glucose level for all patients with diabetes (Note: All blood glucose levels will be performed by the HBO$_2$ staff as close to the initiation of the hyperbaric treatment as possible but not longer than 30 minutes.)

    3.4.6.1 If levels < 90 mg/dL or > 350 mg/dL, notify hyperbaric physician.

    3.4.6.2 Patient may require caloric intake.

    3.4.6.3 Check insulin dose and time.

    3.4.6.4 Check what the patient had to eat and at what time.

3.4.7 Non-insulin dependent diabetics (diet-controlled; no diabetic medications)

    3.4.7.1 Check blood sugar prior to treatment.

    3.4.7.2 If blood sugar greater than 100, begin HBO$_2$ treatment.

    3.4.7.3 If blood sugar less than 100, give glucose/carbohydrate/protein supplementation.

    3.4.7.4 Recheck blood sugar in 15 minutes. (If over 100, begin treatment. If under 100, notify hyperbaric physician for further orders.)

3.4.8 Non-insulin dependent diabetics (oral diabetic medications only):

    3.4.8.1 Check blood sugar prior to treatment.

    3.4.8.2 If blood sugar greater than 110, begin HBO_2 treatment.

    3.4.8.3 If blood sugar less than 110, give glucose/carbohydrate/protein supplementation.

    3.4.8.4 Recheck blood sugar in 15 minutes. (If over 100, begin treatment. If under 110, notify hyperbaric physician for further orders.)

3.4.9 Insulin-dependent diabetics (on ANY type of insulin)

    3.4.9.1 Check blood sugar prior to treatment.

    3.4.9.2 If blood sugar greater than 120, begin HBO_2 treatment.

    3.4.9.3 If blood sugar less than 120, give glucose/carbohydrate/protein supplementation. Record time, amount and type of last insulin injection.

    3.4.9.4 Recheck blood sugar in 15 minutes. (If over 120, begin treatment. If under 120, notify hyperbaric physician for further orders.)

3.4.10 Patients with diabetes should be reminded to notify the hyperbaric nurse at initial onset of signs and symptoms of low blood sugar.

3.4.11 Follow guidelines of the affiliated hospital lab for obtaining blood sugars. Fingers are to be cleaned with nonalcohol swab.

3.5 The hyperbaric physician will be notified of any irregular or abnormal findings and resolve them before the patient is placed in the hyperbaric chamber.

    3.5.1 Check patient for restricted items that are not allowed in the chamber. (Chamber wardrobe should preferably be without pockets.)

    3.5.2 Patient will be grounded via grounding strap for every treatment (Class B chamber).

    3.5.3 Grounding strap will be tested prior to every treatment.

    3.5.4 Patient will demonstrate procedure to clear the ears prior to each treatment.

3.6 The medical record is checked daily for the following:

    3.6.1 New orders

    3.6.2 Lab results, radiology reports, pulmonary function studies, etc. All new findings will be brought to the attention of the hyperbaric physician of record and documented.

3.7 Patients are monitored continuously during the hyperbaric treatment.

    3.7.1 The hyperbaric physician will be immediately available (Class B chamber) and chamber-side (Class A chamber).

    3.7.2 The hyperbaric technician will remain chamber-side for Class B chambers and Class A chambers as well as inside Class A chambers.

3.7.3 The hyperbaric nurse will be immediately available for patient care issues and chamber-side (Class A chamber and Class B) and inside the Class A chamber when appropriate.

3.8 Post-hyperbaric treatment requirements

3.8.1 Blood glucose levels for all patients that have diabetes

3.8.2 Notify hyperbaric physician if blood glucose levels < 90 mg/dL or > 350 mg/dL, or if there is a significant drop during HBO_2 treatment.

3.8.3 Notify patient to check blood glucose levels later in the day. The blood glucose levels have the potential to decrease further.

3.9 Per patient response to HBO_2 treatment

3.9.1 Check ear canals for any changes and record TEED or O'Neill scores when necessary for symptomatic patients or those requiring "stops."

3.9.2 Check lung sounds for any changes.

3.10 Documentation for the hyperbaric treatment to include:

3.10.1 Hyperbaric treatment table utilized

3.10.2 Patient tolerance of hyperbaric treatment

3.10.3 Any adverse events during hyperbaric treatment

3.10.4 Resolution of adverse events

3.10.5 Inside observer(s') time at depth and decompression time, noting repetitive dive group when working inside a Class A chamber

3.10.6 Physician documentation of attendance

407 PATIENT DISCHARGE PLANNING

Purpose

1.1 To establish criteria for patients being discharged from the hyperbaric center

Policy

2.1 The Patient Discharge Plan shall be interdisciplinary and appropriate to the plan of care.

2.2 Patients will be discharged as follows:

    2.2.1 Upon completion of the patient specific treatment plan and have achieved the initial/revised patient specific treatment goals

    2.2.2 When he or she has reached the optimal outcome expected for that patient and return to the care of his or her primary/referring physician

    2.2.3 Patients may/will, at the discretion of the utilization review team of the hyperbaric center, be discharged who are:

        2.2.3.1 Consistently noncompliant with their treatment regime

        2.2.3.2 Consistently fail to keep scheduled appointments

        2.2.3.3 Consistently fail to comply with treatment recommendations

        2.2.3.4 Refuse treatment

Procedure

3.1 Discharge planning will be initiated at the point of entry into the program and shall be completed upon discharge from the center.

3.2 A hyperbaric physician discharge order will be written and documented.

3.3 Discharge instructions to provide continuity shall be communicated to the patient, primary/referring physician, and/or, when appropriate, providers responsible for the patient's continuing health care.

3.4 The nurse case manager shall assess the patient's continued level of understanding of the instructions and document this in the patient record.

3.5 Discharge instruction form will include signatures, date and time.

3.6 Completed Discharge Form

    3.6.1 Original will be put in the patient medical record

    3.6.2 Copy will be given to the patient and/or family

3.7 The office assistant shall accurately maintain a patient discharge report which shall be used to record the patient name and discharged date from the center.

408 HBO₂ SAFETY TIME-OUT STOPS

Purpose

1.1 To enhance safe practice guidelines for patients receiving hyperbaric oxygen treatments

1.2 To be compliant with safety goals

1.3 To combat complacency

Policy

2.1 A safety time-out/pause STOP will be performed prior to the start of every hyperbaric treatment.

Procedures

3.1 A STOP will be completed for Class B monoplace and Class A multiplace chamber operations.

3.2 Two patient identifiers are verified.

3.3 Verify and document

    3.3.1 Right patient

    3.3.2 Right treatment

    3.3.3 Right safety

        3.3.3.1 Patient ground strap (Class B) has been checked prior to every hyperbaric treatment.

        3.3.3.2 Determine all prohibited items are removed from the chamber.

    3.3.4 Patient agreement with treatment or procedure

3.4 The STOP checklist will be dated and signed or initialed by the hyperbaric physician of record and two hyperbaric staff members prior to closing the chamber door and initiating compression.

HYPERBARIC CHAMBER

500 HYPERBARIC CHAMBER MAINTENANCE

Purpose

1.1 To establish guidelines for a safety committee for the hyperbaric center in compliance with NFPA 99-14 (2015)

1.2 Preventive maintenance will be performed on the hyperbaric chamber and related equipment. The forms used for chamber maintenance are specific to chamber manufacturers. Preventive maintenance is performed to reduce the potential for chamber mishaps and patient/staff injury, unplanned repair expenses and loss of revenue due to unexpected chamber shutdown.

Policy

2.1 Hyperbaric chamber and related equipment preventive maintenance must be properly identified, researched, completed, documented and approved by the safety director.

Procedures

3.1 The safety director responsibilities include, but are not limited to, implementation of the safety manual within the hyperbaric center.

    3.1.1 The safety director shall be responsible for regulating all machinery and materials that enter the hyperbaric chamber.

    3.1.2 The safety director shall be responsible for ensuring all preventive maintenance is performed on associated hyperbaric oxygen equipment.

    3.1.3 It is the responsibility of the safety director to ensure all chamber and related equipment checklists are completed and documented at all times.

        3.1.3.1 All forms are verified and signed off by the safety director.

3.2 Preventive Maintenance Schedule

    3.2.1 The Preventive Maintenance Schedule shall be a line-item list of daily, weekly, semiannual, and annual maintenance requirements.

    3.2.2 The Preventive Maintenance Schedule shall be specific for Class A and Class B chambers.

    3.2.3 Line items and periodicities shall be approved of by the hyperbaric safety director. However, any staff member or contractor approved by the hyperbaric safety director may accomplish items within his/her areas of expertise.

    3.2.4 Class B Monoplace

        3.2.4.1 Daily Checklist

            3.2.4.1.1 Mechanical:

                3.2.4.1.1.1 Perform a thorough inspection of the acrylic cylinder or chamber windows.

3.2.4.1.1.2 Inspect chamber door and door-latching mechanism for ease of operation.

3.2.4.1.1.3 Inspect door cam bearing surfaces. (Ensure clean and lightly lubricated.)

3.2.4.1.1.4 Inspect chamber door seal and sealing surfaces.

3.2.4.1.1.5 Inspect inside chamber for cleanliness.

3.2.4.1.1.6 Inspect chamber electrical ground lead for integrity and tight connections.

3.2.4.1.2 Communication System

3.2.4.1.2.1 Check control knobs for security to shaft and ease of operation.

3.2.4.1.2.2 Check for proper communication (i.e. adequate volume and clarity).

3.2.4.1.3 Oxygen

3.2.4.1.3.1 Inspect chamber supply and exhaust hoses (for kinks, loose connections or damage).

3.2.4.1.3.2 Inspect console control knobs and handles for security to shaft and ease of operation.

3.2.4.1.3.3 Ensure that the system on/off switch is in the off position.

3.2.4.1.4 Instruments

3.2.4.1.4.1 Inspect pressure gauges and flow meter for broken lenses or damage.

3.2.4.1.4.2 Inspect both oxygen supply and exhaust bypass indicators in place and undamaged.

3.2.4.2 Weekly Checklists

3.2.4.2.1 Systems (Perform the following operational test with the chamber empty.):

3.2.4.2.1.1 Close and latch chamber door.

3.2.4.2.1.2 Turn the system on/off switch to the "on" position.

3.2.4.2.1.3 Adjust the rate set control to 5.

3.2.4.2.1.4 Adjust the ventilation control for minimum ventilation (fully clockwise).

3.2.4.2.1.5 Adjust pressure set control to 3 psig.

3.2.4.2.1.6 Check to ensure automatic cam locking pin has engaged.

3.2.4.2.1.7 Adjust the pressure set control to 30 psig.

3.2.4.2.1.8 When chamber stabilizes at 3 ATA pressure, readjust the ventilation control (counterclockwise) to 300 lpm. Ensure chamber maintains set pressure while increasing ventilation rate. Readjust ventilation back to minimum rate.

3.2.4.2.1.9 Turn the system on/off switch to the "off" position.

3.2.4.2.1.10 Chamber shall decompress in two minutes or less. Also check that the exhaust bypass indicator is functioning.

3.2.4.2.2 Hyperbaric Chamber

3.2.4.2.2.1 Remove inside rear cover and wipe lint off the exhaust muffler using a clean, dry washcloth.

3.2.4.2.2.2 Ensure rear cover is pushed up against rear head.

3.2.4.2.2.3 Verify weekly continuity reading (ground check) for the system and patient are completed.

3.2.4.2.2.4 Ensure continuity between patient grounding point (wrist strap) and facility ground.

3.2.4.3 Semiannual Checklists

3.2.4.3.1 Hyperbaric Chamber

3.2.4.3.1.1 Compare the chamber pressure gauge and then set pressure gauge for proper calibration. Use the following method to check gauges:

3.2.4.3.1.1.1 Compare gauges when there is zero (0) pressure in chamber and door is open. Both gauges shall read zero (0).

3.2.4.3.1.1.2 When pressurizing chamber, needle movement of both gauges shall be smooth with no hesitation or stepping.

3.2.4.3.1.1.3 If gauges do not operate smoothly, contact chamber manufacturer.

3.2.4.3.1.2 Pressurize the chamber to 30 psig. Leak-check all control and hose connections.

3.2.4.3.1.3 Tighten all connections that leak. If unable to stop leaking, contact safety director and chamber manufacturer.

3.2.4.3.1.4 Inspect treatment chamber and entry lock mufflers.

3.2.4.3.2 Equipment

3.2.4.3.2.1 Remove exhaust mufflers from inside the chamber and clean.

3.2.4.4 Annual Checklists

3.2.4.4.1 Systems

3.2.4.4.1.1 Inspect the chamber relief valve to ensure factory seal is in place. If seal has been disturbed, test relief valve to ensure relief valve is set at 33 psig.

3.2.4.4.1.2 Thoroughly inspect all mechanical systems, including tubing valves and piping for damage or leaks. Make repairs or replace any damaged components.

3.2.4.4.2 Hyperbaric Chamber

      3.2.4.4.2.1 Door and seating surfaces:

            3.2.4.4.2.1.1 Thoroughly clean seal and hatch seating surface.

            3.2.4.4.2.1.2 Inspect sealing surface for any damage or irregularities.

            3.2.4.4.2.1.3 Inspect seal for any damage, hardening or wear.

            3.2.4.4.2.1.4 If seal is free of defects, it shall be thoroughly cleaned, wiped with talc powder, and reinstalled.

    3.2.4.4.2 Perform a thorough visual examination of the internal and external surfaces of the acrylic cylinder for evidence of crazing or physical damage. (Internal baffles/fairings must be removed to provide visual access).

    3.2.4.4.2 If evidence of crazing or damage exists and/or the number of pressure cycles is predicted to exceed the design life before the next annual inspection, it is recommended that the acrylic cylinder be replaced by the chamber manufacturer.

    3.2.4.4.2 Inspect entire chamber system for any deterioration. Note any scratches, nicks, or obvious flaws.

3.3 The checklists for pre- and post-hyperbaric treatments and preventive maintenance are available in the hyperbaric center.

    3.3.1 Daily pretreatment chamber checklist forms will be completed and documented prior to beginning hyperbaric oxygen treatments each morning that patients are treated or before any chamber compression (examples: educational opportunities or testing/maintenance procedures) without patients.

    3.3.2 Post-treatment chamber checklist forms will be completed and documented at the end of each day of hyperbaric oxygen treatments or for chamber compression without patients as above.

    3.3.3 Weekly chamber checklists forms are completed and documented at the end of each week.

    3.3.4 Monthly chamber checklists and preventative maintenance forms are completed and documented monthly.

    3.3.5 Semiannual chamber and related equipment checklists are completed and documented every six months.

    3.3.6 Annual preventive maintenance checklists are completed and documented annually.

3.4 Terms

3.4.1 Preventive Maintenance

Scheduled items of maintenance required to prevent deterioration of the systems from an optimally safe state of readiness.

3.4.2 Corrective Maintenance

Items of maintenance required to return the systems to an optimally safe state of readiness

3.5 Supporting Documents

3.5.1 Systems Deficiency Log

3.5.1.1 The Systems Deficiency Log shall be maintained by the department hyperbaric safety director and utilized by all unit personnel to document any and/or all discrepancies found in the hyperbaric systems and equipment as well as all corrective actions taken. Entries shall include:

3.5.1.1.1 A chronological number

3.5.1.1.2 Date deficiency was discovered

3.5.1.1.3 Description of problem and signature of person who discovered the problem

3.5.1.1.4 Date problem was corrected and signature of person who corrected the problem

3.5.1.1.5 Signature of person who inspected the correction

3.5.1.1.6 Signature of the hyperbaric safety director allowing item back in use

3.5.2 Reentry Control Log

3.5.2.1 The Reentry Control Log shall be maintained by the department hyperbaric safety director and shall contain entries pertinent to all pressure boundaries affecting the hyperbaric systems and subsystems.

3.5.2.2 There must be satisfactory resolutions to any pressure boundary entries PRIOR to any manned chamber runs.

3.5.2.3 The safety director of hyperbaric operations, PRIOR to any manned chamber pressurization, must approve deviation from any complete resolution.

3.5.2.4 Entries shall include:

3.5.2.4.1 A reentry number

3.5.2.4.2 Date problem was discovered

3.5.2.4.3 Description of problem and signature of person who discovered the problem

3.5.2.4.4 Date problem was corrected and signature of person who corrected the problem

3.5.2.4.4.1 Signature of person who inspected the correction

3.5.2.4.5 Signature of the department hyperbaric safety director, or his/her designated appointee

3.5.3 Reentry Control Form

3.4.3.1 The Reentry Control Form shall supplement the Reentry Control Log and shall detail actual work performed. Entries shall include:

3.4.3.1.1 A detailed description of the problem

3.4.3.1.2 The system(s) affected

3.4.3.1.3 The materials needed for the repair

3.4.3.1.4 A detailed description of work performed, tests performed (if necessary), and signature of repairperson

3.4.3.1.5 Signature of inspector

3.4.3.1.6 Signature of department hyperbaric safety director if authorization is necessary to deviate from normal operations

3.6 Class A Multiplace

3.6.1 Mechanical Daily Checklist

3.6.1.1 Open Compressor 1 and Compressor 2 power supply handles.

3.6.1.2 Turn on power to Compressor 1 and Compressor 2.

3.6.1.3 Ascertain the filter gauges read NML (normal).

3.6.1.4 Drain condensation from volume (air handle or receiver) tanks.

3.6.1.5 Verify fire suppression tanks are filled with water and are at appropriate set pressure.

3.6.1.6 Verify all gas cylinders are available, connected and adequately filled with appropriate psi.

3.6.1.7 Check all valves for function and patency.

3.6.1.8 Self-contained breathing apparatus (SCBA) check for appropriate psi and function.

3.6.1.9 Ensure house LOX (liquid oxygen) and VAC (vacuum) lines are opened and functional.

3.6.1.10 Turn on environmental control system if available and ascertain function.

3.6.1.11 All handheld fire hose valves open

3.6.1.12 Suction canister and tubing connected w/Yankauers

3.6.2 Chamber Checklist

3.6.2.1 Evaluate all acrylics for crazing in accordance with ASME/PVHO codes.

3.6.2.2 All chamber lighting is on for all locks.

3.6.2.3 Flow control valves for patient supply closed at each manifold.

3.6.2.4 Exhaust valves on and exhaust flow meter open a quarter of a turn.

3.6.2.5 Breathing apparatus for each occupant in the main lock(s) and transfer (emergency) lock(s), BIBS masks, hoods and tubing

3.6.2.6 BIBS masks tested for proper function.

3.6.2.7 Hearing protection available for all occupants

3.6.2.8 Medical lock (pass through) doors secured inside and out.

3.6.2.9 Transfer (emergency) lock door is secured.

3.6.2.10 Medical equipment such as blood pressure cuff and stethoscope available

3.6.2.11 Blankets and towels available in appropriate number for patients

3.6.2.12 Emergency equipment bag is sealed and not outdated.

3.6.2.13 Oral glucose and fingerstick blood sugar (FSBS) equipment available

3.6.2.14 Sharps container, red bag and emesis basin

3.6.2.15 Fresh drinking water, juice, cups and tissues

3.6.2.16 Non-sterile gloves

3.6.2.17 Spray bottle with fresh water (humidity regulation when necessary)

3.6.2.18 Chamber door ramp up and locked when present prior to assisting patients into the chamber.

3.6.2.19 Communications are all-functioning including speaker system, headset and air phones.

3.6.3 Console/Control Panel/Pretreatment Daily Checklist

3.6.3.1 A/C power turned on

3.6.3.2 CO_2 analyzer on, functional, ready to be calibrated

3.6.3.3 O_2 analyzer on, functional, ready to be calibrated

3.6.3.4 Exhaust valve closed

3.6.3.5 Supply valve open

3.6.3.6 Depth gauges calibrated

3.6.3.7 All panel gauges read appropriate pressure

3.6.3.8 Air to all-line verified

3.6.3.9 Environmental control system (ECS) and fans are on and functional if available.

3.6.3.10 Sample port is open to the oxygen analyzer.

3.6.3.11 Rapid exhaust is closed.

3.6.3.12 Rapid supply is open.

3.6.3.13 Oxygen analyzers are on for all locks and ready to be calibrated when chamber is at treatment depth.

3.6.3.14 CO_2 analyzer for all locks is calibrated to 0.035%.

3.6.3.15 Treatment log and worksheet initiated

3.6.3.16 Patient records are available.

3.6.3.17 Two patient identifiers have been verified and time-out initiated and complete.

3.6.3.18 HBO_2 physician is present for the treatment.

3.6.3.19 Chamber operator, treatment hyperbaric nurse and physician have signed off on appropriate treatment depth and time-out information.

3.6.3.20 Start-up checklist complete.

3.6.3.21 All treatment clocks are synchronized and set to compression depth protocol.

3.6.3.22 All lock lighting set to 70%.

3.6.3.23 Vital signs and blood glucose values complete

3.6.4   Chamber Operator to Inside Observer Checklist

3.6.4.1   Alternate breathing source available for each inside observer (BIBS)

3.6.4.2   Hazardous items check including dentures and hearing aids

3.6.4.3   Hearing protection is on or available for all occupants.

3.6.4.4   Check for repetitive dive profiles for inside observers.

3.6.4.5   Neck rings are on all patients with the supply and exhaust lines attached or BIBS available and functional.

3.6.4.6   There is one hood or BIBS mask per patient.

3.6.4.7   Clamped off all IV and central lines not in use

3.6.4.8   All glass or plastic bottles are vented.

3.6.4.9   Running IVs are noted and if present are free and clear of air; connections are tight and capped.

3.6.4.10 IV drip chamber is to be monitored on descent and ascent.

3.6.4.11 Note the presence of wound VAC devices, hemovacs or suction balls that are open and properly gloved or connected to suction when appropriate.

3.6.4.12 Note any pressure equipment requiring adjustment on ascent or descent.

3.6.4.13 Is the inside observer planning on going above 2000 within 24 hours?

3.6.4.14 Note that the HBO$_2$ physician is present.

3.6.4.15 Treatment protocol verbally confirmed by the physician.

3.6.4.16 Ask for a STOP, STOP, STOP (3X) for any difficulties during descent or ascent.

3.6.4.17 Pretreatment checklist is signed by the chamber operator.

3.6.5   Emergency Treatment Checklist

3.6.5.1   Appropriate medical personnel available

3.6.5.2   ALS pack in chamber

3.6.5.3   Hyperbaric-approved IV pump available and charged

3.6.5.4   Hyperbaric-approved ECG monitor on and ready

3.6.5.5   Breathing circuit connected to hyperbaric approved ventilator

3.6.5.6   Ventilator adjusted by respiratory therapist or physician and tested

3.6.5.7   Spirometer and cuff inflator available

3.6.5.8   IV air precautions checklist complete

3.6.5.9   Suction available and adjusted for chamber pressure

3.6.5.10 Endotracheal tube cuff is filled with saline after removal of air.

3.6.5.11 10 cc syringe and saline available

3.6.5.12 Pressure equipment requiring adjustments on ascent of descent are noted.

3.6.5.13 Inside observers (IO) and chamber operators (CO) signatures

3.6.6   Reach Treatment Depth checklist

3.6.6.1   Patient and inside observers report OK.

3.6.6.2   Treatment breathing gas set to appropriate source.

3.6.6.3   Patients placed on oxygen or breathing gas mixture

3.6.6.4   Chamber ventilation set to appropriate ventilator rate per NFPA guidelines (3 actual cubic feet per minute [ACFM] for all occupants not on BIBS or hoods)

3.6.6.5   Oxygen analyzers calibrated to 20.9%.

3.6.6.6   Complete treatment times and log all occurrences.

3.6.6.7   Notify physician of any occurrences or problems.

POLICY AND PROCEDURAL **GUIDELINES** FOR HYPERBARIC FACILITIES
Copyright © 2017 Best Publishing Company

3.6.6.8 Pressure equipment and drip rates adjusted for treatment pressure.

3.6.6.9 Confirm chamber suction.

3.6.6.10 Chamber operator (CO) initials

3.6.7 Ascent/Leave Bottom Checklist

3.6.7.1 Inside observer and patients off oxygen

3.6.7.2 Lines switched to air or appropriate breathing gas for ascent.

3.6.7.3 Chamber supply is closed off.

3.6.7.4 ECS and fans turned off.

3.6.7.5 Air precautions checklist complete

3.6.7.6 All occupants are ready to ascend.

3.6.7.7 Hyperbaric physician is present and chamber-side.

3.6.7.8 CO initials and signature

3.6.8 Emergency/Transfer Lock Chamber Operator to Inside Observer

3.6.8.1 Hearing protection is on or available.

3.6.8.2 Communications check

3.6.8.3 Hazardous items check

3.6.8.4 Is this an inside observer repetitive dive?

3.6.8.5 Is there a BIBS mask for each occupant available and connected?

3.6.8.6 Is any occupant going above 2000' in the next 24 hours?

3.6.8.7 Are there any glass or plastic bottles that need venting?

3.6.8.8 CO initials and signature

3.7 Class A Multiplace Hyperbaric Chamber and Department Maintenance

3.7.1 Daily Maintenance

3.7.1.1 Wash and disinfect hoods.

3.7.1.2 Disinfect headsets.

3.7.1.3 Clean and disinfect chairs and wipe down chamber floor.

3.7.1.4 Clean the sterile dryer inside and out.

3.7.1.5 Clean BIBS masks.

3.7.1.6 Wipe all patient chairs, door knobs, call bells, and handrails with non-alcohol wipes.

3.7.1.8 Ensure that the lift battery is charged and has been changed weekly.

3.7.2 Weekly Maintenance

3.7.2.1 Log all compressor hours.

3.7.2.2 Log all compressor loads.

3.7.2.3 Clean and maintain console area.

3.7.2.4 Clean all surfaces and chamber chairs.

3.7.2.5 Clean chamber trash cans in and out.

3.7.2.6 Mop main lock and transfer lock floors.

3.7.2.7 Wash/disinfect neck rings and dams.

3.7.2.8 Check compressor cooling oil levels.

3.7.2.9 Clean compressors inside and out.

3.7.2.10 Clean compressor filter mats.

3.7.2.11 Sweep and vacuum compressor room.

3.7.2.12 Check ECS coolant levels.

3.7.2.13 Cycle all chamber valves.

3.7.2.14 Document any changes in the acrylics.

3.7.2.15 Inventory clean supplies.

3.7.3 Semimonthly Maintenance

3.7.3.1 Clean the interiors of all locks.

3.7.3.2 Clean chamber exterior.

3.7.3.3 Vacuum and clean areas under and around the chamber.

3.7.3.4 Clean interior portholes.

3.7.3.5 Clean exterior portholes.

3.7.3.6 Inventory all forms.

3.7.3.7 Clean and organize clean utility room/supply room.

3.7.3.8 Clean and organize the soiled utility room.

3.7.3.9 Clean and organize the storage areas.

3.7.3.10 Prepare equipment bags for new patients.

3.7.3.11 Inspect and clean the hyperbaric stretchers, wheelchairs and removable chairs.

3.7.4 Monthly Maintenance

    3.7.4.1 Calibrate CO monitor.

    3.7.4.2 Calibrate O_2 monitor.

    3.7.4.3 Calibrate CO_2 monitor.

    3.7.4.4 Check all gauges.

    3.7.4.5 Inventory all treatment products.

    3.7.4.6 Review log books and treatment logs for completeness.

    3.7.4.7 Clean and organize all tools and work bench areas.

    3.7.4.8 Inspect chamber O-rings.

    3.7.4.9 Inspect compressor air filters.

3.7.5 Quarterly Maintenance

    3.7.5.1 Inspect and clean regulators.

    3.7.5.2 Check and tighten all BIBS handles.

    3.7.5.3 Check chamber door alignment.

    3.7.5.4 Synchronize all depth gauges.

    3.7.5.5 Test batteries in flashlights and emergency lights.

    3.7.5.6 Clean below deck plates (bilge).

    3.7.5.7 Inspect video cameras.

    3.7.5.8 Inspect and clean headset terminals and plugs.

    3.7.5.9 Inspect all chamber O-rings.

    3.7.5.10 Cycle all chamber valves.

    3.7.5.11 Inspect and clean chamber lighting housings.

    3.7.5.12 Inspect and clean all chamber mufflers.

3.7.6 Semiannual Maintenance

    3.7.6.1 Test fire deluge system.

    3.7.6.2 Sample air receivers.

    3.7.6.3 Leak-test chamber.

    3.7.6.4 Leak-test flexible hoses.

    3.7.6.5 Leak-test all pneumatic actuated valves.

3.7.6.6 Inspect compressor oil filters.

3.7.6.7 Inspect and clean air receivers.

3.7.6.8 Clean ECS heat exchangers.

3.7.6.9 Chamber depressurization test

3.7.6.10 Inspect and clean FSS (fire suppression system) hand-lines, system and storage tank.

3.7.6.11 Check FSS handlines for function.

3.7.6.12 Inspect and lubricate all chamber door O-rings.

3.7.7 Annual Maintenance

3.7.7.1 Chamber air quality test

3.7.7.2 Clean compressor and electrical knife switches for same.

3.7.7.3 Change compressor oil and oil filters.

3.7.7.4 Lubricate door hinge bearings.

3.7.7.5 Realign chamber door hinges.

3.7.7.6 Bench test pressure relief valves or perform pop-off test.

3.7.7.7 Change compressor air filters.

3.7.7.8 Change batteries in patient call bells.

3.7.7.9 Replace O_2, CO_2 and CO sensors.

3.7.7.10 Clean BIBS flow meters and clean and lube flow meter valves.

3.7.7.11 Calibrate all depth gauges and caisson gauges.

3.7.7.12 Calibrate hygrometers.

501 ACRYLIC WINDOW INSPECTION OF CLASS B MONOPLACE AND CLASS A MULTIPLACE

Purpose

1.1 The hyperbaric chamber acrylic window(s) will be inspected each day of chamber operation prior to starting HBO$_2$ therapy and upon completion of HBO$_2$ therapy each day.

1.2 All findings will be documented on the Acrylic Window Inspection Form.

1.3 A continuous record of acrylic window inspections will be maintained within the hyperbaric department.

Policy

2.1 It is strongly suggested that all hyperbaric safety directors be trained in the maintenance and inspection of acrylic windows by taking a course related to these activities.

2.2 Inspection of the acrylic window(s) will assess for damage to allow for repair and to possibly prevent further damage.

Procedure

3.1 The safety director, department director and trained clinicians may/will assist with the inspection.

3.2 It is the responsibility of the safety director to ensure compliance with the inspections.

    3.2.1 Turn on all lighting for best visualization.

    3.2.2 Visually inspect the acrylic windows of the Class A chamber or the tube of the Class B chamber for damage, including:

        3.2.2.1 Crazing

        3.2.2.2 Cracks

        3.2.2.3 Discoloration

        3.2.2.4 Blisters

        3.2.2.5 Scratches

    3.2.3 If no damage, document findings on the Pre/Post-Shift Checklist.

    3.2.4 If damage is noted with the depth of the scratch or pit being 0.01" (the edge of the scratch will catch a fingernail):

        3.2.4.1 Take the chamber out of service.

        3.2.4.2 Document the size and location of the damage. Take a photograph.

        3.2.4.3 Notify the safety director, department director and safety officer.

    3.2.5 Documentation will be included in the hyperbaric chamber log.

502 CLEANING OF HYPERBARIC CHAMBER, RELATED EQUIPMENT AND ROOM

Purpose

1.1 Proper cleaning of equipment reduces the potential for the spread of infection.

1.2 Maintain optimal chamber and related equipment performance.

1.3 Use cleaning product safely in an oxygen-enriched environment.

Policy

2.1 The hyperbaric chamber and related equipment will be cleaned according to:

2.1.1 The type of surface

2.1.2 Potential for equipment damage

2.1.3 Product's compatibility with an enriched oxygen environment

2.1.4 Manufacturer's recommendations

Procedures

3.1 Care and cleaning of chamber, including the acrylic, hyperbaric stretcher and ancillary equipment

3.1.1 Wear gloves at all times when cleaning the hyperbaric chamber and related equipment.

3.1.2 Use the solution per manufacturer's recommendation using a soft, moist cloth.

3.1.2.1 Typically, Tor HB is recommended.

3.1.3 Clean equipment, including the air-break components, between each patient.

3.1.4 The hyperbaric stretcher, mattress and side rails must be cleaned between each patient treatment with the manufacturer's recommended approved solution.

3.1.4.1 Dispose of used sheet, pillow case, gown and blanket in covered linen hamper.

3.1.4.2 Clean stethoscopes, blood pressure cuffs, etc. with above solution between each patient use.

3.1.5 Clean the inside of the chamber at the end of each treatment day with the manufacturer's recommended solution.

3.1.6 At the end of the day, after cleaning the inside (and outside) of the chamber acrylic and related equipment, place the mattress inside the chamber (Class B monoplace).

3.1.7 Clean inside of chamber with manufacturer's recommended solution after treatment when soiled or spills occur.

3.1.8 Clean chamber and related equipment after each treatment for patients with MDROs (multidrug-resistant organisms) or other contaminated drainage.

3.1.9 When scheduling a patient with any MDROs, recommend treating patient at the end of the day.

3.2   General care of equipment

    3.2.1   Always keep the chamber covered with a clean sheet or manufacturer's cover when not in use (Class B monoplace).

    3.2.2   Hyperbaric chamber door is to be kept closed when not in use.

    3.2.3   Do not store items near the hyperbaric chamber that could fall on or against it.

    3.2.4   Do not allow anyone to lean on the hyperbaric chamber.

    3.2.5   Do not allow unauthorized persons or personnel in the chamber area.

    3.2.6   Keep the door to the hyperbaric chamber facility locked when not in use.

3.3   Housekeeping rules regarding cleaning areas in the hyperbaric unit room

    3.3.1   The hyperbaric clinical staff is responsible to clean and maintain the hyperbaric chamber and related equipment as well as the floor surrounding the chamber.

    3.3.2   Housekeeping (facility) staff are responsible to clean the areas away from the hyperbaric chamber and related equipment.

    3.3.3   Housekeeping supervisor is responsible to provide in-services to housekeeping staff regarding restricted cleaning areas in the hyperbaric unit.

    3.3.4   The program director is responsible to ensure the in-service to the housekeeping staff occurs at a minimum of every six months.

503 COMPRESSED GAS CYLINDER, COLOR CODES AND INDEX SYSTEM

Purpose

1.1 To establish guidelines for the color-coding and thread indexing of compressed gas cylinders to reduce the potential for incorrect application or connection

Policy

2.1 Designated clinical personnel shall be familiar and comply with the color-coding of the *Compressed Gas Association Pamphlet C-9 for Medical Gases.*

Procedure

3.1 All medical gases accepted for use at the hyperbaric center shall comply with the color-coding of the *Compressed Gas Association Pamphlet C-9 for Medical Gases.*

3.2 Delivery of compressed gas cylinders not in compliance with the color codes shown herein shall not be accepted.

    3.2.1 If a delivery is accepted and discovered, the cylinders shall be cordoned away from other cylinders and the vendor contacted for immediate removal and replacement with medical gas color-coded cylinders.

3.3 Medical Gas Color-Coding System:

Cylinder Contents	Required Color:
Oxygen	Green
Air	Yellow
Helium	Brown
Heliox	Brown/Green
Nitrogen	Black
Nitrox	Yellow/Green

3.4 Bottled gases or compressed gases all use a thread index system.

    3.4.1 This system is designed to prevent misconnection of cylinders.

    3.4.2 At no time shall anyone modify a gas connection in a manner that shall allow the connection of a gas vessel other than which the system was originally designed.

3.5 The following actions are prohibited:

    3.5.1 Removal or replacement of main cylinder valve

3.5.2 Use of adapters or fittings (Clinical personnel must perform gas analysis/compressed gas safety competency in order to perform required hyperbaric chamber bottled gas connections.)

3.5.3 Painting cylinders so as to change their color

3.6 Only hyperbaric center or medical gas vendor staff that have been trained in this policy shall be permitted to connect cylinders to any bulk or manifold system in the hyperbaric center or department.

3.7 Staff of the hyperbaric center shall be trained in this policy upon hire and annually thereafter.

QUALITY IMPROVEMENT

600 QUALITY IMPROVEMENT

Purpose

1.1 A multidisciplinary approach to gather and review data is utilized to provide optimum outcomes for patients receiving hyperbaric oxygen treatments.

Policy

2.1 The hyperbaric center conducts a monthly ongoing Peer Review/Performance Improvement Program.

2.2 The hyperbaric center participates in the hospital facility Performance/Quality Improvement Plan.

2.3 Quality improvement is a continuous process that involves the entire staff.

2.4 The program director and registered nurse manager are responsible to ensure data elements are in place, reviewed and analyzed per hospital facility guidelines.

Procedure

3.1 Data is gathered to evaluate outcomes to identify areas needing improvement

    3.1.1 By analyzing current performance patterns and trends

    3.1.2 Taking action toward improvement

    3.1.3 Identify and manage sentinel events to reduce the potential for future sentinel events.

3.2 Data will be analyzed on a scheduled basis. The frequency of trending (monthly, quarterly, biannual or annual) and identification is based on the information being trended and hospital policy and schedule recommendations.

3.3 The results of the data analysis are summarized with action plans and follow-up reported at the hospital facility hyperbaric center staff meetings.

3.4 Benchmarks will be established according to best and evidence-based practice of medicine.

601 HYPERBARIC MONTHLY STAFF MEETINGS

Purpose

1.1   To promote communication to the hyperbaric center staff

1.2   To establish standard criteria for monthly staff meetings

Policy

2.1   Staff meetings are to be held monthly.

Procedure

3.1   Hyperbaric center staff meetings are conducted monthly and will/may include but are not limited to the following topics:

    3.1.1 HBO_2 safety issue (Note: Mandatory topic each month)

        3.1.1.1   The safety director is responsible to determine the topic of the month.

    3.1.2   Comprehensive fire drills for HBO_2 to be practiced at least every six months (mandatory)

    3.1.3   Process for patient care issues

    3.1.4   Equipment

    3.1.5   New/revised policies and procedures

    3.1.6   Unit updates and goals

    3.1.7   Infection control and safety measures

    3.1.8   Employee concerns and/or suggestions for improvement

    3.1.9   Quality improvement

3.2   Minutes of staff meetings shall be recorded and available located for easy staff access. These minutes shall include:

    3.2.1   Personnel in attendance and absent

    3.2.2   Topics with discussion of the issues

    3.2.3   Action plan for resolution of identified issues

3.3   Personnel not in attendance are required to read and notate reading.

3.4   Employees are required to attend at least 80% of staff meetings.

3.5   Information between staff meetings may be communicated by

    3.5.1   Written (hard copy or email) memos

    3.5.2   Unit communication book

    3.5.3   Individual and/or group conferences or in-service programs

602 PATIENT CARE CONFERENCES

Purpose

1.1 Patient care conferences are held monthly and may be more frequent as indicated to:

    1.1.1 Facilitate discussion regarding nonhealing patient wounds

    1.1.2 Review/revise the plan of care for continued hyperbaric treatment

    1.1.3 Review patient response to hyperbaric treatment plans

    1.1.4 Discuss dormant (not seen in 30 days or greater) patients and their continued treatment

    1.1.5 Provide transparent communicate to health-care personnel as needed to promote optimal patient outcomes

Policy

2.1 Patient care conferences are held a minimum of monthly to:

    2.1.1. Identify patients that have not progressed according to the current treatment plan

    2.1.2 Review the plan of care and revise as indicated

    2.1.3 Follow-up with appropriate action for optimal patient outcomes

    2.1.4 Follow-up with active patients that have not had contact and/or assessment with the hyperbaric center in 30 days or longer

Procedure

3.1 Team members may include but are not limited to:

    3.1.1. Hyperbaric physicians

    3.1.2 Wound care physicians

    3.1.3 Program director

    3.1.4 Registered nurse manager

    3.1.5 Safety director

    3.1.5 Appropriate clinical staff members

    3.1.6 Patient and family

    3.1.7 Quality improvement (QI) representatives from the hospital

3.2 Discussion includes but is not limited to:

    3.2.1 Dormant/active patients

        3.2.1.1 Program director and nurse manager reviews the patient list to determine current status.

3.2.1.2 If the status unknown, the patient is discussed at the conference with a follow-up letter and/or phone call to the patient and referring physician.

3.2.2 Patients who have not progressed to being healed 50% in 8 weeks

3.2.3 The medical and nursing care plans are updated as indicated with follow-up discussion with the patient and family to determine patient-specific goals.

603 PATIENT AND STAFF SATISFACTION SURVEYS

Purpose

1.1 Hyperbaric patient and staff satisfaction will be evaluated to determine areas for process improvement, identify areas of priorities for patient satisfaction and to promote staff retention.

Policy

2.1 The hyperbaric center will encourage participation in the hospital facility staff and patient satisfaction surveys.

2.2 The hyperbaric center will encourage participation in hyperbaric-specific patient and staff surveys.

2.3 Hyperbaric patient and staff satisfaction surveys will be evaluated quarterly.

Procedure

3.1 The hyperbaric center will participate in hospital facility staff surveys.

3.2 The hyperbaric center will encourage patients to participate in hyperbaric patient satisfaction surveys.

3.3 Patient surveys will contain information on perceptions of care, treatment and services.

3.4 The hyperbaric center will distribute patient satisfaction surveys.

3.5 The collected surveys will be evaluated, then referred to the hospital facility quality improvement committee.

604 INFECTION CONTROL

Purpose

1.1 Standard precautions will be utilized by the hyperbaric staff for any potential or actual exposure to blood or body fluids to decrease the potential for contamination to staff, other patients or visitors.

Policy

2.1 All employees will utilize standard precautions per the hospital facility infection control standards, Center for Disease Control and Prevention (CDC), the State Board of Health, and OSHA (Occupational Safety Health Administration) guidelines.

2.2 The nurse manager has the responsibility to oversee the infection control practice of the hyperbaric center.

    2.2.1 Hyperbaric chambers are to be cleansed at the end of each business day.

    2.2.2 Hyperbaric stretchers are to be cleaned and new linen applied between every patient.

    2.2.3 Hyperbaric chambers are cleaned following any blood or body fluid contamination in the chamber.

    2.2.4 Patients with contaminated draining wounds are typically treated at the end of business day.

2.3 Personnel protective equipment (PPE) will be available and utilized per infection control guidelines.

2.4 Hand washing will be performed per guidelines below.

2.5 Gloves will be utilized for patient contact for blood, body fluids and nonintact skin.

2.6 Waterless, alcohol-based hand rub is NOT allowed in the hyperbaric unit.

2.7 Medications, ointments, creams, etc. that are used from multidose containers will be taken from the container using clean or sterile technique as appropriate for individual use at the patient side. The multidose container will remain at the central storage area.

Procedure

3.1 Personnel protective equipment will be utilized by all employees who have the potential to be exposed to direct blood and body fluids, including nonintact skin and contaminated surfaces.

3.2 Waterless-based hand rub will NOT be utilized when visible contamination of blood and body fluids are observed on the hands.

3.3 Handwashing for all personnel is required at the following times:

    3.3.1 Before and after eating

    3.3.2 After using the restroom

    3.3.3 Before and between patient contact

    3.3.4 Before performing or assisting with procedures

3.3.5 After contact with any body substance or mucous membrane

3.3.6 Before and after contact with wounds

3.3.7 Before, after and when changing gloves

3.3.8 After exposure to surface areas that are contaminated

3.4 Employees are not permitted to eat in work areas.

    3.4.1 Employees working in Class A multiplace chambers are required to stay hydrated throughout the course of the work schedule and should be permitted access to adequate hydration throughout the workday.

3.5 Gloves are to be:

    3.5.1 Worn when coming in contact with contaminated areas

    3.5.2 Changed during patient care when moving from a contaminated site to a clean site

3.6 Handwashing and gloves, using clean or sterile technique as appropriate, will be utilized when removing medications, creams, ointments, etc. from multidose containers.

    3.6.1 Individual doses of medications creams, ointments, etc. will be placed in separate containers and labeled to be taken to patient side for use.

3.7 Artificial fingernails, nail extenders, nail wraps, fresh nail polish or other nail components are not to be worn when providing direct patient care.

3.8 Food and beverages will not be stored in areas where blood or other potentially infectious materials are present.

3.9 Universal precautions will be utilized.

3.10 Isolation techniques will be used per hospital facility policy.

3.11 Recommend ongoing communication with the hospital facility infection control committee as appropriate.

APPENDIX I
Sample Forms for Class A Multiplace and Class B Monoplace Chambers

CHAMBER OPERATOR DAILY START-UP CHECKLIST

Date:

Date	1	2	3	4	5	6	7	8	9	10	11	12	13	14	15	16	17	18	19	20	21	22	23	24	25	26	27	28	29	30	31
Open knife switches for compressors 1 and 2.																															
Drain both volume tanks.																															
Refill trap.																															
Turn on compressor 1.																															
Turn on compressor 2.																															
Check all valves in the mechanical room.																															
CO monitor reads 0ppm.																															
Check water fill level on FS handline tank.																															
O_2 cylinder is open ¼ turn/ record psi.																															
O_2 cylinder del is open ¼ turn/record psi.																															
Air cylinder is open ¼ turn/ record psi.																															
Air del is open ¼ turn /record psi.																															
Check all chamber valves.																															
Turn on main ECS unit.																															
Confirm medical gas & vacuum valves are open.																															

POLICY AND PROCEDURAL GUIDELINES FOR HYPERBARIC FACILITIES
Copyright © 2017 Best Publishing Company

CHAMBER OPERATOR DAILY START-UP CHECKLIST (continued)

Date	1	2	3	4	5	6	7	8	9	10	11	12	13	14	15	16	17	18	19	20	21	22	23	24	25	26	27	28	29	30	31
Check patients' call bells x5.																															
Check air-pak.																															
Check airway box.																															
Turn ML & TL lights on.																															
Turn on AC power.																															
Turn on monitor.																															
Turn on entertainment x2.																															
Turn on fans x2.																															
Turn on ECS x2.																															
Turn on patient monitor screen.																															
Turn on communication box.																															
Cycle TL oxygen, record psi and turn to off position.																															
Cycle TL emergency oxygen, record psi and turn off.																															
Cycle TL air, record psi and leave on.																															
Cycle ML oxygen, record psi and turn off.																															
Cycle ML emergency O₂, record psi and turn off.																															

Date	1	2	3	4	5	6	7	8	9	10	11	12	13	14	15	16	17	18	19	20	21	22	23	24	25	26	27	28	29	30	31
Cycle ML air, record psi and leave on.																															
Record psi for FSS deluge.																															
Record psi for FSS handline.																															
Compressor psi is greater than 150.																															
Both ML depth gauges are at 0 FSW.																															
Both TL depth gauges are at 0 FSW.																															
O_2 analyzers are on x3.																															
CO_2 analyzer is on and calibrated.																															
Sound-powered phone is functioning.																															
ML supply and exhaust valves closed.																															
TL supply and exhaust valves are closed.																															
Rapid exhaust is closed; supply rapid closure open.																															
Check temp monitoring system for alerts. Report to nurse manager.																															
Technicians' initials x2 and time																															

POLICY AND PROCEDURAL **GUIDELINES** FOR HYPERBARIC FACILITIES
Copyright © 2017 Best Publishing Company

MAINTENANCE FORM SAMPLES

WEEKLY MAINTENANCE (Initial and Date)				
	WEEK 1	WEEK 2	WEEK 3	WEEK 4
Clean Console; Wipe Down All Surfaces				
Clean All Surfaces of Chamber Chairs				
Clean Metal Trash Cans in Chamber Inside and Out				
Wash and Disinfect Neck Rings and Dams; Dust And Lube				
Inspect Cooling Oil Levels of Compressors				
Clean Compressors Inside and Out with a Damp Cloth				
Change Compressors' Filter Mats				
Sweep and Vacuum Mechanical Room				
Check Antifreeze/Coolant Level in the ECS				
Cycle Transfer Lock and Main Lock Valves				
Inspect Portholes and Document Changes				
*** Inventory Supplies in Clean and Soiled Utility Room				

MAINTENANCE FORM SAMPLES (continued)

SEMIMONTHLY MAINTENANCE (Initial And Date)				
	WEEK 1	WEEK 2	WEEK 3	WEEK 4
Clean All Surfaces Inside the Main Lock and Transfer Lock				
Clean Medical Lock's Interior				
Dust and Damp Mop Chamber Exterior				
Vacuum Under and Around the Chamber				
Clean Interior Portholes				
*** Clean Exterior Portholes				
***Inventory All Forms; Print As Needed				
***Clean and Organize Clean Utility Room				
*** Clean and Organize Soiled Utility Room				
*** Clean and Organize Storage Room				
*** Prepare Equipment Bags for New Patients				
Clean and Disinfect Hyperbaric Stretcher and Wheelchair, and After Each Use				

MONTHLY MAINTENANCE (Initial and Date)	
Calibrate CO Monitor	
Calibrate O_2 Monitor	
Complete Monthly Gauge Log	
*** Inventory Oxygen Breathing Products	
*** Inspect Logbook and Treatment Sheets	
***Organize Workbench and Tool Box	
Inspect Chamber O-Rings	
Inspect Compressor Air Filters	
Inspect SCBA and Smoke Hoods	

MAINTENANCE FORM SAMPLES (continued)

Department of Hyperbaric Medicine Maintenance Record

MONTH: April   YEAR: _____

MAINTENANCE	WEEK 1	WEEK 2	WEEK 3	WEEK 4
Compressor #1 Hours				
Compressor #1 Load				
Compressor #2 Hours				
Compressor #2 Load				

DAILY MAINTENANCE	WEEK 1				WEEK 2				WEEK 3				WEEK 4			
Wash and Disinfect Hoods																
Disinfect Headsets																
Clean/Disinfect Chairs and Wipe Down Floor in Main Lock																
Clean Sterile Drier Inside and Out																
Clean BIBS Masks																
*** Wipe All Patient Chairs, Door Knobs, Call Bells, and Handrails with Non-Alcohol Wipes																

MAINTENANCE FORM SAMPLES (continued)

WEEKLY MAINTENANCE (Initial and Date)				
	WEEK 1	WEEK 2	WEEK 3	WEEK 4
Clean Console; Wipe Down All Surfaces				
Clean All Surfaces of Chamber Chairs				
Clean Metal Trash Cans in Chamber Inside and Out				
Wash and Disinfect Neckrings and Dams/Dust and Lube				
Inspect Cooling Oil Levels of Compressors				
Clean Compressors Inside and Out with a Damp Cloth				
Change Compressors' Filter Mats				
Sweep and Vacuum Mechanical Room				
Check Antifreeze/Coolant Level in the Ecs				
Cycle Transfer Lock and Main Lock Valves				
Inspect Portholes and Document Changes				
*** Inventory Supplies in Clean and Soiled Utility Rooms				

POLICY AND PROCEDURAL **GUIDELINES** FOR HYPERBARIC FACILITIES
Copyright © 2017 Best Publishing Company

MAINTENANCE FORM SAMPLES (continued)

SEMIMONTHLY MAINTENANCE (Initial and Date)				
	WEEK 1	WEEK 2	WEEK 3	WEEK 4
Clean All Surfaces Inside the Main Lock and Transfer Lock				
Clean Medical Lock's Interior				
Dust and Damp Mop Chamber Exterior				
Vacuum Under and Around the Chamber				
Clean Interior Portholes				
*** Clean Exterior Portholes				
***Inventory All Forms; Print As Needed				
***Clean and Organize Clean Utility Room				
*** Clean and Organize Soiled Utility Room				
*** Clean and Organize Storage Room				
*** Prepare Equipment Bags for New Patients				
Clean and Disinfect Hyperbaric Stretcher and Wheelchair After Each Use				

MAINTENANCE FORM SAMPLES (continued)

MONTHLY MAINTENANCE (Initial and Date)	
Calibrate CO Monitor	
Calibrate O_2 Monitor	
Complete Monthly Gauge Log	
*** Inventory Oxygen-Breathing Products	
*** Inspect Logbook and Treatment Sheets	
***Organize Workbench and Tool Box	
Inspect Chamber O-Rings	
Inspect Compressor Air Filters	
Inspect SCBA and Smoke Hoods	

MONTHLY MAINTENANCE SPECIFIC TO APRIL (Initial and Date)	
Clean Regulators/Inspect Parts	
Inspect All BIBS Handles; Tighten As Needed	
Snoop Flexible Hoses	
Sample Air in Holding Tanks	

MAINTENANCE FORM SAMPLES (continued)

INITIALS	PRINT NAME	SIGNATURE

MAINTENANCE FORM SAMPLES (continued)

Department of Hyperbaric Medicine Maintenance Record

MONTH: August   YEAR: _____

MAINTENANCE	WEEK 1	WEEK 2	WEEK 3	WEEK 4
Compressor #1 Hours				
Compressor #1 Load				
Compressor #2 Hours				
Compressor #2 Load				

DAILY MAINTENANCE	WEEK 1						WEEK 2						WEEK 3						WEEK 4					
Wash and Disinfect Hoods																								
Disinfect Headsets																								
Clean/Disinfect Chairs and Wipe Down Floor in Main Lock																								
Clean Sterile Drier Inside and Out																								
Clean BIBS Masks																								
*** Wipe All Patient Chairs, Door Knobs, Call Bells, and Handrails with Non-Alcohol Wipes																								

MAINTENANCE FORM SAMPLES (continued)

WEEKLY MAINTENANCE	WEEK 1	WEEK 2	WEEK 3	WEEK 4
Clean Console				
Clean All Surfaces of Chamber Chairs				
Clean Chamber Trash Cans				
Mop Mainlock and Transfer Lock Floors				
Wash/Disinfect Neckrings and Dams				
Check Compressors' Cooling Oil Levels				
Clean Compressors Inside and Out				
Clean Compressors' Filter Mats				
Sweep and Vacuum Compressor Room				
Check ECS Coolant Level				
Cycle All Chamber Valves				
Document Any Changes in the Acrylics				
*** Inventory Supplies in Clean Utility Room				

MAINTENANCE FORM SAMPLES (continued)

SEMIMONTHLY MAINTENANCE				
	WEEK 1	WEEK 2	WEEK 3	WEEK 4
Clean Interior of Main Lock and Transfer Lock				
Clean Medical Lock				
Clean Chamber Exterior				
Vacuum and Clean Areas Under and Around the Chamber				
Clean Interior Portholes				
*** Clean Exterior Portholes				
***Inventory All Forms				
***Clean/Organize Clean Utility Room				
*** Clean/Organize Soiled Utility Room				
*** Clean/Organize Storage Room				
*** Prepare Equipment Bags for New Patients				
***Inspect and Clean Hyperbaric Stretcher and Wheelchair				

MAINTENANCE FORM SAMPLES (continued)

MONTHLY MAINTENANCE	
Calibrate CO Monitor	
Calibrate O_2 Monitor	
Calibrate CO_2 Monitor	
***Check All Gauges	
*** Inventory Oxygen-Breathing Products	
*** Review Logbook and TX Sheets	
***Clean and Organize Tools and Work Bench	
Inspect Chamber O-Rings	
Inspect Compressor Air Filters	

MONTHLY MAINTENANCE SPECIFIC TO AUGUST (Initial and Date)	
Align Chamber Door and Hatches, and Inspect Hinges during Annual Maintenance	
Inspect Fire Suppression Handlines	
Clean FSS Handline Storage Tank. Inspect Interior Tank	
Test Pressure Relief Valves during Annual Maintenance	
Calibrate All Ml and Tl Depth Gauges (Annual Maintenance)	
Replace O_2 Sensors and Calibrate	

MAINTENANCE FORM SAMPLES (continued)

INITIALS	PRINT NAME	SIGNATURE

MAINTENANCE FORM SAMPLES (continued)

MONTHLY MAINTENANCE SPECIFIC TO DECEMBER (Initial and Date)	
Clean Headset Terminals and Plugs	
Examine Compressors' Oil Filters	
Clean Chamber Lights (Housing)	
Clean All Chamber Mufflers	

MAINTENANCE FORM SAMPLES (continued)

Department of Hyperbaric Medicine Maintenance Record

MONTH: January YEAR: _____

MAINTENANCE	WEEK 1	WEEK 2	WEEK 3	WEEK 4
Compressor #1 Hours				
Compressor #1 Load				
Compressor #2 Hours				
Compressor #2 Load				

DAILY MAINTENANCE	WEEK 1							WEEK 2							WEEK 3							WEEK 4						
Wash and Disinfect Hoods																												
Disinfect Headsets																												
Clean/Disinfect Chairs and Wipe Down Floor in Main Lock																												
Clean Sterile Drier Inside and Out																												
Clean BIBS Masks																												
*** Wipe All Patient Chairs, Door Knobs, Call Bells, and Handrails with Non-Alcohol Wipes																												

MAINTENANCE FORM SAMPLES (continued)

WEEKLY MAINTENANCE	WEEK 1	WEEK 2	WEEK 3	WEEK 4
Clean Console				
Clean All Surfaces of Chamber Chairs				
Clean Chamber Trash Cans				
Mop Mainlock and Transfer Lock Floors				
Wash/Disinfect Neckrings and Dams				
Check Compressors' Cooling Oil Levels				
Clean Compressors Inside and Out				
Clean Compressors' Filter Mats				
Sweep and Vacuum Compressor Room				
Check ECS Coolant Level				
Cycle All Chamber Valves				
Document Any Changes in the Acrylics				
*** Inventory Supplies in Clean Utility Room				
Inspect Chamber O-Rings				

MAINTENANCE FORM SAMPLES (continued)

SEMIMONTHLY MAINTENANCE				
	WEEK 1	WEEK 2	WEEK 3	WEEK 4
Clean Interior of Main Lock and Transfer Lock				
Clean Medical Lock				
Clean Chamber Exterior				
Vacuum and Clean Areas Under and Around the Chamber				
Clean Interior Portholes				
*** Clean Exterior Portholes				
***Inventory All Forms				
***Clean/Organize Clean Utility Room				
*** Clean/Organize Soiled Utility Room				
*** Clean/Organize Storage Room				
*** Prepare Equipment Bags for New Patients				
***Inspect and Clean Hyperbaric Stretcher and Wheelchair				

MAINTENANCE FORM SAMPLES (continued)

MONTHLY MAINTENANCE	
Calibrate CO Monitor	
Calibrate O_2 Monitor	
Calibrate CO_2 Monitor	
***Check All Gauges	
*** Inventory Oxygen-Breathing Products	
*** Review Logbook and TX Sheets	
***Clean and Organize Tools and Work Bench	
Lube Chamber O-Rings If Needed	
Inspect Compressor Air Filters	

MONTHLY MAINTENANCE SPECIFIC TO JANUARY (Initial and Date)	
Clean Regulators/Examine Parts	
Examine BIBS Handles; Tighten As Needed	
Inspect Flashlight Batteries in Chamber	
Inspect Video Cameras	
Snoop Chamber Penetrators at 165 FSW	
Rapid Decompression Test from 165 FSW	
Clean Compressor Knife Switches	
Check SCBA and Smoke Hoods	

MAINTENANCE FORM SAMPLES (continued)

INITIALS	PRINT NAME	SIGNATURE

MAINTENANCE FORM SAMPLES (continued)

Department of Hyperbaric Medicine Maintenance Record

MONTH: March   YEAR: _____

MAINTENANCE	WEEK 1	WEEK 2	WEEK 3	WEEK 4
Compressor #1 Hours				
Compressor #1 Load				
Compressor #2 Hours				
Compressor #2 Load				

DAILY MAINTENANCE	WEEK 1							WEEK 2							WEEK 3							WEEK 4						
Wash and Disinfect Hoods																												
Disinfect Headsets																												
Clean/Disinfect Chairs and Wipe Down Floor in Main Lock																												
Clean Sterile Drier Inside and Out																												
Clean BIBS Masks																												
***Wipe All Patient Chairs, Door Knobs, Call Bells, and Handrails with Non-Alcohol Wipes																												

MAINTENANCE FORM SAMPLES (continued)

WEEKLY MAINTENANCE	WEEK 1	WEEK 2	WEEK 3	WEEK 4	WEEK 5
Clean Console					
Clean All Surfaces of Chamber Chairs					
Clean Chamber Trash Cans					
Mop Main Lock and Transfer Lock Floors					
Wash/Disinfect Neckrings and Dams					
Check Compressors' Cooling Oil Levels					
Clean Compressors Inside and Out					
Clean Compressors' Filter Mats					
Sweep and Vacuum Compressor Room					
Check ECS Coolant Level					
Cycle All Chamber Valves					
Document Any Changes in the Acrylics					
Inventory Supplies Clean Utility Room					

MAINTENANCE FORM SAMPLES (continued)

SEMIMONTHLY MAINTENANCE				
	WEEK 1	WEEK 2	WEEK 3	WEEK 4
Clean Interior of Main Lock and Transfer Lock				
Clean Medical Lock				
Clean Chamber Exterior				
Vacuum and Clean Areas Under and Around the Chamber				
Clean Interior Portholes				
*** Clean Exterior Portholes				
***Inventory All Forms				
***Clean/Organize Clean Utility Room				
*** Clean/Organize Soiled Utility Room				
*** Clean/Organize Storage Room				
*** Prepare Equipment Bags for New Patients				
***Inspect and Clean Hyperbaric Stretcher and Wheelchair				

MAINTENANCE FORM SAMPLES (continued)

MONTHLY MAINTENANCE	
Calibrate CO Monitor	
Calibrate O_2 Monitor	
Calibrate CO_2 Monitor	
Check All Gauges	
*** Inventory Oxygen-Breathing Products	
*** Review Logbook and TX Sheets	
***Clean and Organize Tools and Work Bench	
Inspect Chamber O-Rings	
Inspect Compressor Air Filters	

MONTHLY MAINTENANCE SPECIFIC TO MARCH (Initial and Date)	
Clean Headset Terminals and Plugs	
Examine Compressors' Oil Filters	
Clean Housings for Chamber Lighting	
Clean All Chamber Mufflers	
Clean Bilge	
Test Fire Suppression Deluge System	
Lubricate Door and Hatch Hinges	
Calibrate Hygrometer	

MAINTENANCE FORM SAMPLES (continued)

INITIALS	PRINT NAME	SIGNATURE

MAINTENANCE FORM SAMPLES (continued)

MONTHLY MAINTENANCE SPECIFIC TO SEPTEMBER (Initial and Date)	
Clean Headset Terminals and Plugs	
Inspect Compressor Oil Filters	
Inspect and Clean Chamber Lighting Housing	
Inspect and Clean All Chamber Mufflers	
Clean Bilge	
Test Fire Deluge System	
Compressor Annual Maintenance Performed	

MONTHLY MAINTENANCE SPECIFIC TO OCTOBER (Initial and Date)	
Clean Regulators/Inspect Parts	
Check BIBS Handles; Tighten As Needed	
Snoop All Flexibile Hoses for Leaks	
Sample Air in Holding Tanks	
Check SCBA and Smoke Hoods	

MONTHLY MAINTENANCE SPECIFIC TO JUNE (Initial and Date)	
Examine Compressor Oil Filters	
Clean Housing of Chamber Lighting	
Clean Headset Terminals and Plugs	
Clean All Chamber Mufflers	

MAINTENANCE FORM SAMPLES (continued)

Department of Hyperbaric Medicine Maintenance Record

MONTH: May   YEAR: _____

MAINTENANCE	WEEK 1	WEEK 2	WEEK 3	WEEK 4	WEEK 5
Compressor #1 Hours					
Compressor #1 Load					
Compressor #2 Hours					
Compressor #2 Load					

DAILY MAINTENANCE	WEEK 1					WEEK 2					WEEK 3					WEEK 4				
Wash and Disinfect Hoods																				
Disinfect Headsets																				
Clean/Disinfect Chairs and Wipe Down Floor in Main Lock																				
Clean Sterile Drier Inside and Out																				
Clean BIBS Masks																				
*** Wipe All Patient Chairs, Door Knobs, Call Bells, and Handrails with Non-Alcohol Wipes																				

MAINTENANCE FORM SAMPLES (continued)

WEEKLY MAINTENANCE	WEEK 1	WEEK 2	WEEK 3	WEEK 4	WEEK 5
Clean Console					
Clean All Surfaces of Chamber Chairs					
Clean Chamber Trash Cans					
Mop Main Lock and Transfer Lock Floors					
Wash/Disinfect Neckrings and Dams					
Check Compressors' Cooling Oil Levels					
Clean Compressors Inside and Out					
Clean Compressors' Filter Mats					
Sweep and Vacuum Compressor Room					
Check ECS Coolant Level					
Cycle All Chamber Valves					
Document Any Changes in the Acrylics					
*** Inventory Supplies in Clean Utility Room					

MAINTENANCE FORM SAMPLES (continued)

SEMIMONTHLY MAINTENANCE					
	WEEK 1	WEEK 2	WEEK 3	WEEK 4	WEEK 5
Clean Interior of Main Lock and Transfer Lock					
Clean Medical Lock					
Clean Chamber Exterior					
Vacuum and Clean Areas Under and Around the Chamber					
Clean Interior Portholes					
***Clean Exterior Portholes					
***Inventory All Forms					
***Clean/Organize Clean Utility Room					
***Clean/Organize Soiled Utility Room					
***Clean/Organize Storage Room					
***Prepare Equipment Bags for New Patients					
Inspect and Clean Hyperbaric Stretcher and Wheelchair					

MAINTENANCE FORM SAMPLES (continued)

MONTHLY MAINTENANCE	
Calibrate CO Monitor	
Calibrate O_2 Monitor	
Calibrate CO_2 Monitor	
Check All Gauges	
*** Inventory Oxygen-Breathing Products	
*** Review Logbook and TX Sheets	
***Clean and Organize Tools and Work Bench	
Inspect Chamber O-Rings	
Inspect Compressor Air Filters	

MONTHLY MAINTENANCE SPECIFIC TO MAY (Initial and Date)	
Check Chamber Door Alignment	
Clean ECS Heat Exchangers	

MAINTENANCE FORM SAMPLES (continued)

INITIALS	PRINT NAME	SIGNATURE

MONTHLY MAINTENANCE SPECIFIC TO NOVEMBER	
Check Alignment of Chamber Door and Hatches	
Clean ECS Heat Exchangers	

PRETREATMENT CHECKLIST

Inside Observer (IO) :

- Metal clipboard, pad of paper, and pen.
- Hood supply valves closed at each manifold.
- Exhaust valves on and exhaust flow open a ¼ turn for each patient.
- Scott masks x7 in ML and TL; test for function.
- Breathing equipment for each patient: neck rings, hoods, and tubing.
- Hearing protection for each IO and patient.
- Transfer lock door securely closed.
- BVMs available; masks filled with saline, tubing and adapter.
- Stethoscope and blood pressure cuffs x2.
- Emergency bag sealed. Check inventory sheet for expiration dates.
- 3 finger stick bags and 3 tubes of glutose; check expiration dates.
- Blankets and towels stocked.
- S, M, L non-sterile gloves on shelf by TL.
- Drinking water, juice, cups, and tissues.
- TL hand held fire hose valve is open.
- Red bags, emesis basin and sharps container
- TL suction canister connected to tubing with yankauer.
- S, M, L non-sterile gloves on shelf by ML.
- ML hand held fire hose valve is open.
- ML suction canister connected to tubing with yankauer.
- Medlock door secured inside and out.
- Inspect portholes for TX 1. Report findings to the safety director. N/A
- Spray bottle with warm water for humidity. N/A
- Raise the ramp to the chamber door. N/A

IOs' initials: _____

Emergency Pretreatment Checklist: N/A

- Suitable medical and technical staff available.
- Orange emergency pack in chamber, sealed.
- Pressure bag available for IV fluids.
- Suction available.
- Sterile normal saline IV flushes available.
- Foley catheter balloon inflated with normal saline solution.
- Air and IV precaution checklist complete.

Initials: _____

Emergency Checklist at Depth: N/A

- Patients and IO(s) report okay.
- Patients on 100% oxygen via hood.
- Confirm chamber suction.
- Pressure equipment and IV drip rates adjusted.
- Oxygen analyzers calibrated to 20.9%.
- Chamber vent set at 3acfm for each occupant not breathing oxygen.
- Complete treatment times, and log all data and events.
- Physician notified of any incidents.

CO initials: _____

At Depth Checklist:

- Patients and IO(s) report okay.
- Patients on 100% oxygen via hood
- Pressure equipment adjusted
- O_2 analyzer calibrated to 20.9%
- Chamber vent set at 3acfm for each occupant not breathing oxygen.
- Complete treatment times, and log all data and events.
- Physician notified of any incidents.

CO initials: _____

PRETREATMENT CHECKLIST (continued)

Chamber Operator (CO):	Leave Bottom Checklist:
o CO startup checklist completed with initials x2 and time.	o Patients and IO(s) off oxygen and ready to ascend.
o ML and TL lights on.	o Chamber supply closed and ML treatment gas switched to air.
o ML and TL treatment gases switched to air.	o ECS and fans off x2.
o All console gauges display appropriate psi.	o Air precautions checklist complete.
o Sample port open for oxygen analyzer.	o HBO$_2$ physician present.
o Oxygen analyzers turned on x3	CO initials: _____
o Carbon dioxide analyzer on and calibrated to 0.035%.	
o Console clocks synchronized and timers set for treatment protocol.	**Transfer Lock Checklist: N/A**
o ECS and fans on x2.	o Communication system works.
o Fill out log book and treatment worksheet.	o Are you happy with the transfer lock?
o Patients' records, vital signs, and blood glucose are available.	o Is this an IO repetitive dive?
o Blood glucose recorded on the treatment sheets.	o Hearing protection is on.
o Two patient identifiers (name and date of birth) have been verified.	o Hazardous items check.
CO's initials: _____ RN's initials: _____	o Bibs masks are set up for at least 3 IOs.
	o IO going over 2000 feet in the next 24 hours.
	o Glass or plastic bottles that need to be vented.
	CO initials: _____

POLICY AND PROCEDURAL GUIDELINES FOR HYPERBARIC FACILITIES
Copyright © 2017 Best Publishing Company

PRETREATMENT CHECKLIST (continued)

CO to IO:

o   Communication system works.

o   Are you happy with the chamber?

o   Do you have a BIBS mask for each IO?

o   Have you checked for hazardous items on patients and self?

o   Hearing protection is on or available?

o   Is this an IO repetitive dive?

o   Neck rings are on patients with supply and exhaust lines attached and there is one hood per patient.

Air Precautions:

o   Central lines and heplocks not in use are clamped.

o   Glass and plastic bottles are vented.

o   Wound vacuums, hemovacs and suction balls are open.

o   Pressure equipment requiring adjustment.

IV Precautions:

o   Any running IVs. N/A

   o   IV lines free of air

   o   IV connections tight and capped

   o   Drip chamber must be monitored on ascent and descent

o   IO(s) going above 2,000 feet in the next 24 hours.

o HBO_2 physician is present.

o   Patient treatment protocol verified by physician.

o   Ask for a stop 3 times for any problem.

CO initials: _____

Initials	Signature	Date/Time

HBO_2 physician present during hyperbaric treatment:

_____

Signature   Date/ Time

U.S. NAVY TREATMENT TABLE 9

Dive # _____   Date: _____

LS _____ 0 FSW   RS _____ 0 FSW

	30 Minute O₂ Session	5 Minute Air Break	30 Minute O₂ Session	5 Minute Air Break	30 Minute O₂ Session	

RB _____ 45 FSW   LB _____ 45 FSW
   On O₂   Off O₂   On O₂   Off O₂   On O₂   Off O₂

20 Minute O₂ Session	5 Minute Air Break	20 Minute O₂ Session	5 Minute Air Break	20 Minute O₂ Session	5 Min. Air Break	20 Minute O₂ Session

Off O₂   On O₂   Off O₂   On O₂   Off O₂   On O₂   Off O₂

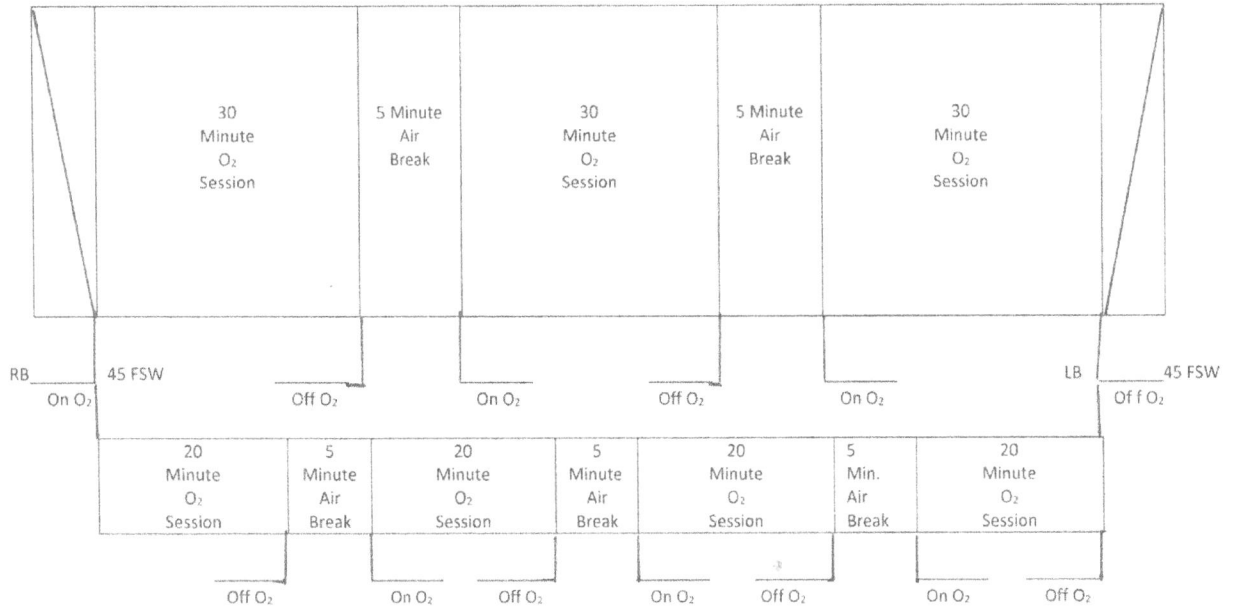

Compression   Decompression
Rate: ft. /min.   Rate: ft. / min.
: 10 /:15 /:___   :10 /:15 /: ___

Team Member	Patient Name	MR#	Tx #	IP/OP	BG		Stops	#1	#2
CO#1	1						Pt #		
CO#2	2						Direction		
IO#1	3						Depth		
IO#2	4						Stops	#3	#4
IO#3	5						Pt #		
IO#4	6						Direction		
RN	7						Depth		
Physician	8						Stops	#5	#6
Physician	9						Pt #		
	10						Direction		
	11						Depth		
	12								

Schedules	IO#1	IO#2	IO#3	IO#4	Chamber	Cycles:	Additional Information:
LS						ML:	
RS							
TBT							
TDT						TL:	
TTD							
Schedule							
RGD						MDLK:	
Max Depth							

APPENDIX II
Acronyms

AGE	Arterial Gas Embolism	**LB**	Left Bottom
ASME	American Society of Mechanical Engineers	**LP**	Low Pressure
ASTM	American Society for Testing and Materials	**LPM**	Liters per Minute
ATA	Atmosphere Absolute	**LS**	Left Surface
ATP	Ambient Temperature and Pressure	**MBC**	Maximal Breathing Capacity
BCLS	Basic Cardiac Life Support	**MCC**	Main Control Console
BIBS	Built-In Breathing System	**MD**	Maximum Depth
BNA	Baromedical Nurses Association	**MDR**	Medical Device Reporting
BNACB	Baromedical Nurses Association Certification Board	**MEV**	Manual Exhaust Valve
		MIFR	Maximum Inspiratory Flow Rate
BPM	Breaths per Minute	**ML**	Main lock
BVM	Bag Valve Mask	**MSW**	Meters of Sea Water
CGA	Compressed Gas Association	**MVV**	Maximum Ventilatory Volume
CNS	Central Nervous System	**NBDHMT**	National Board of Diving and Hyperbaric Medical Terminology
CPR	Cardiopulmonary Resuscitation		
DAN	Divers Alert Network	**NITROX**	Nitrogen-Oxygen
DCS	Decompression Sickness	**NFPA**	National Fire Protection Association
DT	Dive Time or Descent Time	**NOAA**	National Oceanic and Atmospheric Administration
DT/DG	Dive Timer/Depth Gauge		
EBA	Emergency Breathing Apparatus	**NO-D**	No Decompression
ECS	Environmental Control System	**OBD**	Overboard Dump
EGS	Emergency Gas Supply	**O&M**	Operating and Maintenance
ENT	Ear, Nose, and Throat	**OPs**	Operating Procedures
EPs	Emergency Procedures	**OSHA**	Occupational Safety and Health Administration
FDA	Food and Drug Administration		
FFM	Full Face Mask	**PMS**	Planned Maintenance System
FFW	Feet of Freshwater	**PNS**	Peripheral Nervous System
FPM	Feet per Minute	**POS**	Person on the Spot
FSS	Fire Suppression System	**PP**	Partial Pressure
FSW	Feet of Seawater	**PPCO$_2$**	Partial Pressure Carbon Dioxide
HBO$_2$	Hyperbaric Oxygen	**PPM**	Parts per Million
IL	Inner Lock	**PPO$_2$**	Partial Pressure Oxygen
IO	Inside Observer (tender)	**PSI**	Pounds per Square Inch

PSIA Pounds per Square Inch Absolute

PSIG Pounds per Square Inch Gauge

PVHO Pressure Vessels for Human Occupancy

QA Quality Assurance

QI Quality Improvement

RB Reached Bottom

RMV Respiratory Minute Ventilation

RNT Residual Nitrogen Time

ROV Remotely Operated Vehicle

RQ Respiratory Quotient

RS Reached Surface

RSP Render Safe Procedure

SAD Safe Ascent Depth

SCA System Certification Authority

SCBA Self Contained Breathing Apparatus

SCF Standard Cubic Feet

SCFM Standard Cubic Feet per Minute

SCFR Standard Cubic Feet Required

SCUBA Self-Contained Underwater Breathing Apparatus

SDS Saturation Diving System

SET Surface Equivalent Table

SEV Surface Equivalent (percent or pressure)

SI Surface Interval or System International

SLED Sea Level Equivalent Depth

SLM Standard Liters per Minute (short version used in formulas)

SLPM Standard Liters per Minute

STP Standard Temperature and Pressure

SUR D Surface Decompression

SUR D AIR Surface Decompression Using Air

SUR D O$_2$ Surface Decompression Using Oxygen

TBT Total Bottom Time

TDT Total Decompression Time

TJC The Joint Commission

TL Transfer Lock

TLC Total Lung Capacity

TLV Threshold Limit Values

TM Technical Manual

TMDER Technical Manual Deficiency Evaluation Report

TRC Transportable Recompression Chamber

TRCS Transportable Recompression Chamber System

TTD Total Time of Dive

UBA Underwater Breathing Apparatus

UHMS Undersea and Hyperbaric Medical Society

REFERENCES

1. Moon RE. Air or gas embolism. In: Weaver LK, editor. Undersea and Hyperbaric Medical Society. Hyperbaric oxygen therapy indications. 13th ed. Best Publishing Co.; 2014. p. 1-9.

2a. Murphy-Lavoie H, Butler F, Hagan C. Central retinal artery occlusion. In: Weaver LK, editor. Undersea and Hyperbaric Medical Society. Hyperbaric oxygen therapy indications. 13th ed. Best Publishing Co.; 2014. p. 11-23.

2b. Worth ER, Tettelbach WH, Hopf HW. Enhancement of healing in selected problem wounds. In: Weaver LK, editor. Undersea and Hyperbaric Medical Society. Hyperbaric oxygen therapy indications. 13th ed. Best Publishing Co.; 2014. p. 25-56.

3. Weaver LK. Carbon monoxide poisoning. In: Weaver LK, editor. Undersea and Hyperbaric Medical Society. Hyperbaric oxygen therapy indications. 13th ed. Best Publishing Co.; 2014. p. 47-65.

4. Bakker DJ. Clostridial myonecrosis (gas gangrene). In: Weaver LK, editor. Undersea and Hyperbaric Medical Society. Hyperbaric oxygen therapy indications. 13th ed. Best Publishing Co.; 2014. p. 67-75.

5. Baynosa RC, Zamboni WA. Compromised grafts and flaps. In: Weaver LK, editor. Undersea and Hyperbaric Medical Society. Hyperbaric oxygen therapy indications. 13th ed. Best Publishing Co.; 2014. p. 77-90.

6. Strauss MB. Crush injuries and skeletal muscle-compartment syndromes. In: Weaver LK, editor. Undersea and Hyperbaric Medical Society. Hyperbaric oxygen therapy indications. 13th ed. Best Publishing Co.; 2014. p. 91-103.

7. Moon RE. Decompression sickness. In: Weaver LK, editor. Undersea and Hyperbaric Medical Society. Hyperbaric oxygen therapy indications. 13th ed. Best Publishing Co.; 2014. p. 105-12.

8. Feldmeier JJ. Delayed radiation injuries (soft tissue and bony necrosis). In: Weaver LK, editor. Undersea and Hyperbaric Medical Society. Hyperbaric oxygen therapy indications. 13th ed. Best Publishing Co.; 2014. p. 113-37.

9. Piper SM, Murphy-Lavoie H, LeGros TL. Idiopathic sudden sensorineural hearing loss. In: Weaver LK, editor. Undersea and Hyperbaric Medical Society. Hyperbaric oxygen therapy indications. 13th ed. Best Publishing Co.; 2014. p. 139-51.

10. Barnes RC. Intracranial abscess. In: Weaver LK, editor. Undersea and Hyperbaric Medical Society. Hyperbaric oxygen therapy indications. 13th ed. Best Publishing Co.; 2014. p. 153-7.

11. Jacoby I. Necrotizing soft tissue infections. In: Weaver LK, editor. Undersea and Hyperbaric Medical Society. Hyperbaric oxygen therapy indications. 13th ed. Best Publishing Co.; 2014. p. 159-77.

12. Hart BB. Refractory osteomyelitis. In: Weaver LK, editor. Undersea and Hyperbaric Medical Society. Hyperbaric oxygen therapy indications. 13th ed. Best Publishing Co.; 2014. p. 179-207.

13. Van Meter KW. Severe anemia. In: Weaver LK, editor. Undersea and Hyperbaric Medical Society. Hyperbaric oxygen therapy indications. 13th ed. Best Publishing Co.; 2014. p. 209-15.

14. Cianci P, Slade JB Jr, Sato RM, Faulkner J. Thermal burns. In: Weaver LK, editor. Undersea and Hyperbaric Medical Society. Hyperbaric oxygen therapy indications. 13th ed. Best Publishing Co.; 2014. p. 217-38.

15. Guidelines for: standards of care for the patient receiving hyperbaric oxygen therapy (HBO$_2$) [Internet]. Baromedical Nurses Association. Available from: http://hyperbaricnurses.org/about-us/standards-of-care/

RESOURCES

2016 Ambulatory care accreditation overview: a snapshot of the accreditation process [Internet]. The Joint Commission. 12 p. Available from: https://www.jointcommission.org/assets/1/18/AHC_Overview_Guide_2016.pdf

2017 National Patient Safety Goals [Internet]. 1 screen. Available from: https://www.jointcommission.org/standards_information/npsgs.aspx

American Society of Mechanical Engineers. Safety standard for pressure vessels for human occupancy: in-service guidelines. PVHO-2-2012 ed. ASME; 2012.

Burman F. Risk assessment guide for installation and operation of clinical hyperbaric facilities. 5th ed. San Antonio (TX): International ATMO, Inc.; 2015. Ref. 1.6.1-1.6.21.

Burman F, Sheffield R, Posey K. *Decision process to assess medical equipment for hyperbaric use.* Undersea Hyperb Med. 2009; Mar-Apr;36(2):137-44.

CGA G-4.3-2007 Commodity specification for oxygen. 6th ed. Compressed Gas Association.

Clinical hyperbaric facility accreditation manual [Internet]. 2005 ed. rev. 1. Dunkirk (MD): Undersea and Hyperbaric Medical Society, Inc.; 2005. 83 p. Available from: https://www.uhms.org/images/Accreditation-Documents/2005_accreditation_manual__r.pdf

Crouch MJ. How administration affects facility safety. In: Workman T, editor. Hyperbaric facility safety: a practical guide. Flagstaff (AZ): Best Publishing Co.; 2002. p. 710-11.

Kindwall EP. Contradictions and side effects to hyperbaric oxygen treatment. In: Kindwall EP, Whelan HT, editors. Hyperbaric medicine practice. 3rd ed. Flagstaff (AZ): Best Publishing Co.; 2008. p. 273-88.

Larson-Lohr V, Norvell H, Josefsen L, Wilcox JR, editors. Hyperbaric nursing and wound care. Flagstaff (AZ): Best Publishing Co.; 2010.

Manufacturer and User Facility Device Experience Database - (MAUDE) [Internet]. U.S. Food and Drug Administration (FDA). Available from: https://www.fda.gov/medicaldevices/deviceregulationandguidance/postmarketrequirements/reportingadverseevents/ucm127891.htm

McGinn-Merritt W, Skarban M. Hyperbaric nursing education. In: Larson-Lohr V, Norvell HC, editors. Hyperbaric nursing. Flagstaff (AZ): Best Publishing Co.; 2002. p. 351-9.

McHowell W. Care of the patient receiving hyperbaric oxygen therapy. In: Larson-Lohr V, Norvell HC editors. Hyperbaric nursing. Flagstaff (AZ): Best Publishing Co.; 2002. p 134-143.

Messina VJ, Norkool DM. Hyperbaric nursing. In: Kindwall EP, Whelan HT, editors. Hyperbaric medicine practice. 3rd ed. Flagstaff (AZ): Best Publishing Co.; 2008. p. 227-44.

Miller LM, Josefsen L. Staff competency and training. In: Larson-Lohr V, Norvell H, Josefsen L, Wilcox JR. editors. Hyperbaric nursing and wound care. Flagstaff (AZ): Best Publishing Co.; 2010. p 191-197.

National Board of Diving & Hyperbaric Medical Technology [Internet]. Columbia (SC): National Board of Diving and Hyperbaric Medical Technology; c2001-2017. NBDHMT recommended guidelines for clinical internship in HBO technology. Available from: http://www.nbdhmt.org/index.asp

NFPA 99: Health care facilities code. 2015 ed. National Fire Protection Association; 2015. Chapter 14, Hyperbaric facilities.

Norvell H, Larson-Lohr V, Fabus S, Josefsen L. Patient education. In: Larson-Lohr V, Norvell HC, editors. Hyperbaric nursing. Flagstaff (AZ): Best Publishing Co.; 2002. p.244-5.

O'Neill OJ, Weitzner ED. The O'Neill grading system for evaluation of the tympanic membrane: A practical approach for clinical hyperbaric patients. Undersea Hyperb Med. 2015; May-Jun;42(3):265-71.

Technical Committee on Hyperbaric and Hypobaric Facilities (HEA-HYP) Memorandum [Internet]. 2012 Jul. 29 p. Available from: https://www.nfpa.org/Assets/files/AboutTheCodes/99/99_HEA-HYP_A2014_FDAgenda_8-12.pdf

Undersea & Hyperbaric Medical Society [Internet]. North Palm Beach (FL): Undersea and Hyperbaric Medical Society. Safety time out/pause – "stop"; 2014 Jul; [about 1 screen]. Available from: https://www.uhms.org/resources/news-announcements/106-safety-time-out-pause-stop-posted-7-31-2014.html

Undersea & Hyperbaric Medical Society [Internet]. North Palm Beach (FL): Undersea and Hyperbaric Medical Society. MEDFAQs: Do you have to attend a safety director course to be a safety director of a hyperbaric program? In other words, is attending the course a recognized standard?; 2015 Jul 7; [about 1 screen]. Available from: https://www.uhms.org/resources/medfaqs-frequently-asked-questions-faq/search/1-%20Search.html?yrfaqsearch=safety

United States Department of Labor, Occupational Safety and Health Administration [Internet]. Washington (DC): Occupational Safety and Health Administration. Hazard communication standard: safety data sheets [about 8 screens]. Available from: https://www.osha.gov/Publications/OSHA3514.html

U.S. Navy diving manual. Rev. 6. Washington (DC): U.S. Government Printing Office; 2008.

Vincent HG. Documentation of the nursing process as it relates to hyperbaric oxygen therapy. In: Larson-Lohr V, Norvell HC editors. Hyperbaric nursing. Flagstaff (AZ): Best Publishing Co.; 2002. p 85-94.

Workman W. How to manage your hyperbaric facility safety program. In: Workman W, editor. Hyperbaric facility safety: a practical guide. Flagstaff (AZ): Best Publishing Co.; 2010. p. 638-9.

Workman W. How to manage your hyperbaric facility safety program. In: Hyperbaric nursing. Larson-Lohr V, Norvell HC, editors. Flagstaff (AZ): Best Publishing Co.; 2002. p. 298-300.

UNITED STATES DEPARTMENT OF LABOR, Occupational Safety and Health Administration [Internet]. Washington (DC): Occupational Safety and Health Administration. Hazard communication standard: safety data sheets [about 8 screens]. Available from: https://www.osha.gov/Publications/OSHA3514.html

INDEX

A

abscess 25, 30, 145

acidosis 40

accreditation agencies 17

acrylic window inspection
    iv, 91

administration iii, v, 12, 14, 42,
    65, 101, 142, 147-148

air breaks iv, 26, 30, 42, 65,
    68, 71

air embolism 54

anemia 26, 30, 145

antibiotics 31

anxiety. *See also* confinement
    anxiety iii, 38, 43, 48-49

appendix iv, 103, 141

arterial insufficiencies 25, 28

arterial lines 5

atmospheric pressure 9

B

barotrauma iii, 37-38, 45-47, 63,
    68

billing iii, 17, 60, 62

blood glucose iii, 41-43, 51-52,
    73, 75, 85

BNA iii, 72, 142

BNACB 6, 10

board certification 9-10

bomb threat iii, 55-56

burns 26, 145

C

carbon monoxide poisoning 25-
    26, 145

cell phone. *See also* electronic
    devices iii, 59

central retinal artery 25, 28, 145

checklists. *See also* forms 66,
    78-81

chokes 28

Class A chamber. *See also*
    multiplace chamber 6, 9-10,
    20, 27, 36-39, 42-44, 46, 48-49,
    55, 68, 72, 74-75, 91

Class B chamber. *See also*
    monoplace chamber 9, 36-
    37, 42, 44, 46, 48, 55, 74, 91

claustrophobia. *See also*
    confinement anxiety iii, 38,
    48

clinical research. *See also* research
    iii, 13

clinical studies 25

clostridial myonecrosis 25, 145

clostridial myositis 26

communication 1, 4, 6, 19, 21, 36,
    49, 63-64, 73, 79, 97, 102, 148

confinement anxiety iii, 38, 48-49

consent iv, 13, 17, 19, 48, 62-63,
    65-66, 72

contraindications iii, 5, 53

crush injury 27

D

debridement 30-31, 63

decompression 10, 20, 25, 27-28,
    35-39, 41-44, 55-57, 68, 75,
    142-143, 145

decompression sickness 10, 25,
    27-28, 41, 142, 145

delayed radiation injury 31

diabetes 20, 29, 41-42, 51-52,
    72-75

diving 6, 28, 45, 142-143, 147-
    148

documentation iii, iv, 9, 17, 19,
    21, 68-70, 72, 75, 91, 148

E

education iii, ix, 1-3, 5, 9-12, 14, 18,
    20, 46, 64, 72, 147-148

electronic devices. *See also* cell
    phone iii, 59

embolism 25-26, 37, 41, 54, 142,
    145

    gas embolism 25-26, 41, 142,
        145

emergency iii, v, 23, 32-33, 36-37,
    39, 43-44, 49, 55, 84, 86-87,
    89, 142

environment 1-3, 8-9, 14, 24, 32,
    43, 48, 53, 58, 92

equipment iv, 3, 5, 7, 9, 14, 18, 23,
    26, 33-34, 36, 55-56, 58, 64,
    66, 78, 80-82, 84, 86-88, 92-
    93, 97, 101, 147

    clean 92

    emergency 84

eustachian tube dysfunction
    45-46, 68

F

fire 8, 33-36, 39, 63-64, 66-67, 73,
    83, 89-90, 97, 142, 147

fluorescein angiogram 29

food 102, 142, 147

forms. *See also* checklist iv, v, 23,
    62, 78, 81, 88, 103

free radicals 54

G

gases 27, 94

gas gangrene 25-26, 31, 145

grafts 25, 27, 31, 145

H

hours of operation 6

HBO$_2$ iii, iv, 1, 3, 5-6, 13, 17, 19,
    26-33, 41-49, 51-52, 54, 58,
    64-68, 70-75, 77, 85-86, 91,
    97, 142, 145

hyperbaric oxygen iii, iv, ix, 1-3,
    5-6, 8, 17, 19, 25-26, 29-31,
    40-42, 45, 48, 51, 53-54, 57,
    59-61, 63, 65-66, 70-73, 77-78,
    81, 96, 142, 145, 147-148

hyperbaric oxygen therapy ix, 2-3,
    5, 8, 19, 25-26, 29, 31, 40, 45, 48,
    57, 60-61, 63, 72, 145, 147-148

hypoglycemia 41, 52, 72

I

incident reports iii, 23

infection iv, 3, 24, 45, 53, 92, 97,
    101-102

    control iv, 3, 24, 97, 101-102

www.ingramcontent.com/pod-product-compliance
Lightning Source LLC
Chambersburg PA
CBHW081537220326
41598CB00036B/6470